D1526516

Alternatives to Animal Testing

Edited by Christoph A. Reinhardt

On behalf of the Swiss Institute for
Alternatives to Animal Testing, SIAT

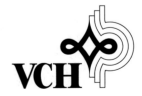

© VCH Verlagsgesellschaft mbH, D-69451 Weinheim (Federal Republic of Germany), 1994

Distribution:
VCH, P. O. Box 101161, D-69451 Weinheim, Federal Republic of Germany
Switzerland: VCH, P. O. Box, CH-4020 Basel, Switzerland
United Kingdom and Ireland: VCH, 8 Wellington Court, Cambridge CB1 1HZ, United Kingdom
USA and Canada: VCH, 220 East 23rd Street, New York, NY 10010–4606, USA
Japan: VCH, Eikow Building, 10-9 Hongo 1-chome, Bunkyo-ku, Tokyo 113, Japan

ISBN 3-527-30043-0 (VCH, Weinheim)   ISBN 1-56081-831-X (VCH, New York)

Alternatives to Animal Testing

New Ways in the Biomedical Sciences, Trends and Progress

Edited by
Christoph A. Reinhardt

On behalf of the Swiss Institute for
Alternatives to Animal Testing, SIAT

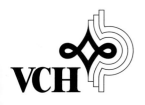

VCH

Weinheim · New York
Basel · Cambridge · Tokyo

Editor:
Dr. C. A. Reinhardt
SIAT
Swiss Institute for Alternatives to Animal Testing
Technopark, Pfingstweidstr. 30
CH-8005 Zürich

Published jointly by
VCH Verlagsgesellschaft mbH, Weinheim (Federal Republic of Germany)
VCH Publishers Inc., New York, NY (USA)

Editorial Director: Dr. Hans F. Ebel
Production Manager: Dipl.-Wirt.-Ing. (FH) H.-J. Schmitt

Library of Congress Card No.: applied for

British Library Cataloguing-in-Publication Data:
A catalogue record for this book
is available from the British Library

Die Deutsche Bibliothek – CIP-Einheitsaufnahme:
Alternatives to animal testing : new ways in the biochemical sciences,
trends and progress / ed. by Christoph A. Reinhardt.
– Weinheim ; New York ; Basel ; Cambridge ; Tokyo :
VCH 1994
   ISBN 3-527-30043-0
NE: Reinhardt, Christoph A. [Hrsg.]

Composition: Hagedornsatz, D-68519 Viernheim
Printing: betz-druck, D-64291 Darmstadt
Bookbinding: J. Schäffer, D-67269 Grünstadt
Printed in the Federal Republic of Germany.

Preface

When I moved into the field of alternatives to animal testing, only a few people foresaw how rapidly this field would develop in the following 10 to 15 years. Two of them, Richard Steiner and Gerhard Zbinden, agreed in 1981 to launch my first three-year project on in vitro cytotoxicity as a replacement of in vivo experiments. This agreement was made possible by the equally farsighted president and staff of the Foundation FFVFF (Fonds für versuchstierfreie Forschung, Zürich), in particular through Ms. Irène Hagmann who acted as a most diplomatic mediator between these two exponents of divergent positions on animal experimentation at that time. Mr. Steiner was the patron of the project as president of the Swiss Animal Protection (SAP) organization (Schweizer Tierschutz, STS). Professor Zbinden, as director of the Institute of Toxicology of the Swiss Federal Institute of Technology (ETH) and the University of Zurich, acted as host and scientific supervisor of my project. At that time, he always insisted on not using the word "alternatives," but he fully supported the idea and the scientific concept of in vitro technologies as the basis of all in vitro alternatives to animal testing. Although Steiner and Zbinden often held diametrically opposing views on animal experimentation, our joint project opened many minds for constructive dialogue and factually correct discussions on a politically – and at that time almost exclusively emotionally argued – sensitive issue. Because of their input into the development of alternatives, I invited both of them to be Guests of Honor at the symposium on *Alternatives to Animal Testing,* held at the ETH Zurich on the 30th of November in 1992.

Leading scientists and key promoters of the field of alternatives to animal testing, such as Andrew Rowan, Oliver Flint, Michael Balls and Horst Spielmann, were invited to contribute as speakers to that symposium together with other active researchers. About 170 participants assembled in Zurich and were welcomed on behalf of the recently founded Swiss Institute for Alternatives to Animal Testing, SIAT. The Organizing Committee included members of the faculty of the Swiss Federal Institute of Technology (Max Dobler, Ulrich Müller-Herold and Friedrich Würgler) and Sergio Bellucci of the Management and Technology Institute at Technopark Zurich, who together with his staff superbly managed the practical details of this successful symposium. In his opening address, the Vice President for Research of the ETH, Ralf Hütter, pointed out the necessity of searching for new alternatives to animal testing. At the same time, he underlined the importance of basic biomedical research at the ETH as well as in other research institutions world wide, with its implications for the use of and experimentation on at least some live animals. He acknowledged that the approaches presented at the symposium were certainly appropriate to the goal of improving animal well-being. In closing the symposium, Hans-Peter Schreiber (the newly elected deputy for ethics at the ETH) appealed to the audience to promote shifts from our traditional anthropocentric view to a more balanced understanding of animals which currently are used or abused.

The present volume contains the main presentations made at this symposium, carefully reviewed and updated to include developments up to fall 1993.

In the introductory chapter, Andrew Rowan looks back over the *33 years since Russell and Burch invented the Three Rs: Refine, Reduce, Replace.* Having been part of the original scene at FRAME in England, he eventually ended up at Tufts University near Boston where he became the first director of the Center for Animals and Public Policy (CAPT). He strongly influenced public policy in the early "Draize Campaign," which was most successful (in the U.S.) in starting the search for replacements of the Draize eye irritation test in a number of large companies in the cosmetics industry.

Hugo Van Looy, from the OECD headquarters in Paris where he is responsible for the field of chemical safety, describes Three Rs developments in the context of *international regulatory acceptance.* The OECD guidelines involving animal testing contain method descriptions for toxicity testing without prescribing their use for regulatory acceptance (for which only national or EC regulatory authorities are competent). They do, however, have a major influence on the selection of "necessary tests," and for that reason the role of the OECD headquarters in evaluating *refine/reduce alternatives* is important. More recently, this development has been shifted towards *replace alternatives* by the new head of the Chemical Safety Commission, Hermann Koëter (the former chairman of the European Research Group for Alternatives to Animal Testing, ERGATT).

The European Centre for the Validation of Alternative Methods (ECVAM) is the constructive result of years of discussion at the two EC Directorate Generals XI and XII. At the symposium in November 1992, the interim director Erminio Marafante described the plans and infrastructure of the center. In April 1993, Michael Balls, who had most efficiently promoted alternatives to animal testing as chairman of the trustees of FRAME in England, was appointed director of the center. Because he has already very actively taken up his duties at ECVAM in Ispra, his most recent plans have also been included in the last section of this chapter (Chap. 3).

The *timetable for replacing, reducing and refining animal use* can certainly be accelerated *with the help of in vitro tests,* as Oliver Flint eloquently and competently outlines in chapter 4. As an industrial toxicologist he has always actively promoted in vitro test procedures within his company (and formerly at ICI in England) and at national and international gatherings. His outline of the time course of the development, validation and acceptance of the Limulus amebocyte lysate (LAL) test might be a cautious warning for those who think that alternatives to animal testing are easily produced and quickly accepted by regulatory authorities.

In the first chapter on national activities, the *Fund for the Replacement of Animals in Medical Experiments (FRAME)* and its *23 years of campaigning for the Three Rs* is impressively described by Michael Balls and Julie Fentem. Michael Balls' initiative and influence have brought FRAME to its current position of world leadership in promoting the field of alternatives, and his activities are respected in industry and academia as well as in animal protection circles. His recent move to ECVAM to assume European leadership of alternatives was the logical step for him and a wise selection by the responsible authorities of the EC.

The next two chapters are about recent developments in the Netherlands.

As the veterinarian responsible for the animal facility of the University of Utrecht, Bert van Zutphen documents the development of *animal use and alternatives* in his country. He has actively promoted refine and reduce aspects of alternatives and will be host and key organizer of the 2nd World Congress of Alternatives and Animal Use in 1996. He describes the recent creation of a national research center for alternatives in Utrecht. At the *RIVM (National Institute of Public Health and Environmental Protection) Center for Alternatives to Animal Testing* the concept of *the Three Rs* is being implemented *in quality control of vaccines.* Coenraad Hendriksen describes his scientific approach using biochemical assays as alternatives in the area of potency testing and quality control of vaccines, where almost all animal testing is seriously discomforting.

Within only three years, *ZEBET, the national German Center for Documentation and Evaluation of Alternatives to Animal Experiments at the Federal Health Office (BGA) in Berlin,* has been developed by its director, Horst Spielmann, into one of the leading institutions in the field. ZEBET's most recent success is the regulatory acceptance of the Hen's Egg Test (HET-CAM) as a routine test for screening corrosive chemicals. The German *databank for alternatives to animal experiments of the Akademie für Tierschutz,* the so-called "Yellow List," is described in chapter 9 by Brigitte Rusche and Ursula Sauer.

The Swiss Institute for Alternatives to Animal Testing, SIAT, was founded in 1991 on the initiative of Angelo Vedani and myself, now the scientific directors of their respective research groups. I have described the *SIAT research, teaching and consulting program in the area of in vitro toxicology* in chapter 10, and work in the field of *computer-aided drug design and the Three Rs* is presented in chapter 11 by Vedani.

Chapter 12 contains an overview on *computer-aided programs in biomedical education,* attractively written and illustrated by the veterinarian Richard Fosse, who encourages the use of such programs by his students and experimental scientists as alternatives in his laboratory animal facility in Bergen, Norway.

The next six chapters describe various fields of activities and detailed research projects as examples of the widespread interdisciplinary character of alternatives to animal testing. The educational project *TEMPUS* is outlined by the participating European partners (Miroslav Červinka and others, chapter 13). In the area of parasitology, the *replacement of laboratory animals in the management of blood-sucking arthropods* (chapter 14 by Achim Issmer and coworkers) and the *maintenance of filarial cycles in the laboratory* (chapter 15 by Joachim Rapp and coworkers) are current topics of development and progress. New techniques for improving the drug metabolizing capacity of hepatocytes co-cultured with other epithelial cells are described by Rolf Gebhardt in chapter 16. The characterization and use of long-term liver cultures to evaluate bone marrow toxicity is explained by Brian Naughton and coworkers (chapter 17). A European interlaboratory evaluation of a new in vitro ocular irritation model is presented by Peter Joller and coworkers in chapter 18. And finally, Mary Dawson and Zara Jabar describe their cellular assays for testing peritoneal dialysis plastic bags (chapter 19).

The last chapter rounds this volume off with a surprisingly provocative position taken by the Swiss regulatory authorities. Lavinia Pioda is responsible for regulating toxic chemicals at the Federal Health Office in Bern. She has critically followed the development of alternatives over the past decades and has always – in contrast to the regulatory authorities of some larger countries – followed a very open policy for new methods aimed at decreasing the requirements for animal testing. She sees the development of alternatives to animal testing as a revolution in our approach to testing in general, calling not only for new methodologies but for new ways of thinking.

Acknowledgements. Ms. Bonnie Strehler receives my warmest thanks for her most competent and efficient help in reviewing, correcting and formatting the chapters of this book. She also translated a part of the manuscripts into American English to give the book a homogeneous style. The interest and agreeable collaboration of Dr. Hans F. Ebel of the VCH Verlagsgesellschaft in Weinheim is gratefully acknowledged. Last, but not least, I would like to thank the Swiss pharmaceutical companies, Ciba-Geigy, F. Hoffmann-La Roche AG, and Sandoz Pharma AG, for their generous financial support.

Zurich, October 7, 1993   Christoph A. Reinhardt

IN MEMORIAM

Sadly enough, the death of Professor Gerhard Zbinden on the 28th of September, 1993, in Vienna brought to a close the life of an influential scientist and active promoter of in vitro toxicology. His foreword was to have appeared on this page. Instead, I would like to dedicate this book to his memory.

Christoph A. Reinhardt

Foreword

From the perspective of a comprehensive ethical animal protection, and as former President of the World Society for the Protection of Animals, WSPA, I offer my congratulations on the realization of this exceptional book. I am surprised and gratified by the documentation made available of international developments in the field of alternatives to animal testing – alternatives which are worthy of the name, although, of course, the replacement of animals in testing is a special concern of mine.

The predominance of the natural sciences in our time has hardly been favorable to this development. On the contrary, it has been the work of a few dedicated researchers – most of whom have contributed to this book – who have shown courage and perseverance not only in developing new scientific methods but also in establishing the appropriate infrastructures. Their efforts have led to the development of an international network of activities which continually attracts new researchers. As a result, a genuinely interdisciplinary, ethically oriented science has come into being which is truly unique.

In the past decades, experts from the universities and industry, from governmental agencies and animal protection quarters have often disagreed about the definition and the "right" objectives of alternatives to animal testing. Complementary methods, supplementary or adjunct methods, alternative methods, in vitro technology, or simply better basic research – why all the bother? What really counts in every instance is the Three Rs. Whether it is a question of an application for the approval of an experiment using animals, the planning of an animal experiment, or the search for methods for the development of a better medication, the number of animals used will be reduced, fewer animals will be subjected to stressful procedures or irreversibly damaged, and above all, fewer animals will be sacrificed. Fewer and fewer laboratory mice, rats, rabbits, dogs, cats, and other domestic animals, but also primates: this is the decisive point in judging the quality of alternative methods.

We have come surprisingly far in this period. Awareness of alternatives has reached the highest circles of the OECD and the EG, and in many instances these methods are already being evaluated. This book should contribute not only to a wider recognition of the developments which have already taken place in the field of alternatives but also to the advancement of alternative methods in the future. I express my appreciation to the contributors and wish the book its due success.

Zurich, October 4, 1993

Richard Steiner
Past President of the World Society
for the Protection of Animals

List of contributors

Prof. Dr. M. Balls
ECVAM
JRC Environment Institute
I-21020 Ispra (Varese)
Italy

Dr. M. Červinka
Charles University Medical Faculty
Department of Biology
Simkova 870
50038 Hradec Králové
Czech Republic

Dr. Z. Červinková
Charles University Medical Faculty
Department of Physiology
Simkova 870
50038 Hradec Králové
Czech Republic

Dr. A. Coquette
Laboratoires J. Simon
Vieux Chemin du Poète 10
B-1301 Wavre
Belgium

Dr. M. Dawson
Department of
Pharmaceutical Sciences
University of Strathclyde
Glasgow G1 1WX
Scotland

Dr. J. H. Fentem
FRAME
34 Stoney Street
Nottingham NG1 1NB
England

Dr. O. Flint
In Vitro Toxicology
Bristol-Myers Squibb
P.O. Box 4755
Syracuse, NY 13221
USA

Dr. R. T. Fosse
Laboratory Animal Veterinary
Services
Biomedical Research Center
University of Bergen
N-5021 Bergen
Norway

Prof. Dr. R. Gebhardt
Physiologisch-chemisches Institut
der Universität
Hoppe-Seyler-Strasse 4
D-72076 Tübingen
Germany

Dr. B. Grune-Wolff
ZEBET
Robert von Ostertag Institut
des BGA
Postfach 480 447
D-12254 Berlin
Germany

Dr. hab. J. Grunewald
Institute of Tropical Medicine
University of Tübingen
Wilhelmstrasse 27
D-72074 Tübingen
Germany

Dr. C. F. M. Hendriksen
National Institute of Public Health
and Environmental Protection
P.O. Box 1
3720 BA Bilthoven
The Netherlands

W. H. Hoffmann
Institute of Tropical Medicine
University of Tübingen
Wilhelmstrasse 27
D-72074 Tübingen
Germany

A. E. Issmer
Institute of Tropical Medicine
University of Tübingen
Wilhelmstrasse 27
D-72074 Tübingen
Germany

Dr. Z. Jabar
Department of Pharmaceutical
Sciences
University of Strathclyde
Glasgow G1 1WX
Scotland

Dr. P. W. Joller
ANAWA Laboratories Inc.
CH-8602 Wangen
Switzerland

L. Keller
Institute of Tropical Medicine
University of Tübingen
Wilhelmstrasse 27
D-72074 Tübingen
Germany

Dr. H. B. W. M. Koëter
OECD Environment Directorate
2 rue André Pascal
F-75775 Paris
France

Dr. M. Liebsch
ZEBET
Robert von Ostertag Institut
des BGA
Postfach 480 447
D-12254 Berlin
Germany

Dr. P. K. Logemann
Advanced Tissue Sciences, Inc.
10933 North Torrey Pines Rd.
LaJolla, CA 92037-1005
USA

Dr. E. Marafante
ECVAM
JRC Environment Institute
I-21020 Ispra (Varese)
Italy

Dr. B. A. Naughton
Advanced Tissue Sciences, Inc.
Hematology Laboratory
505 Coast Blvd. South
LaJolla, CA 92037
USA

Dr. G. K. Naughton
Advanced Tissue Sciences, Inc.
Hematology Laboratory
505 Coast Blvd. South
LaJolla, CA 92037
USA

Dr. J. Noben
Janssen Biotech N. V.
Lammerdries 55
B-2250 Olen
Belgium

Dr. L. Pioda
Bundesamt für Gesundheitswesen
Abteilung Gifte
Bollwerk 27
Postfach 2644
CH-3001 Bern
Switzerland

Dr. R. Pirovano
Istituto di Richerche Biomediche
"A. Marxer" RBM S.p.A.
Via Carpaccio 8
I-20133 Milano
Italy

J. Rapp
Institute of Tropical Medicine
University of Tübingen
Wilhelmstrasse 27
D-72074 Tübingen
Germany

Dr. C. A. Reinhardt
Swiss Institute for Alternatives
to Animal Testing (SIAT)
Technopark
Pfingstweidstrasse 30
CH-8005 Zurich
Switzerland

Prof. Dr. A. Rowan
Center for Animals
and Public Policy
School of Veterinary Medicine
Tufts University
200 Westboro Road
N. Grafton, MA 01536
USA

Dr. B. Rusche
Akademie für Tierschutz
Spechtstrasse 1
D-85579 Neubiberg
Germany

Dr. J. San Román
Advanced Tissue Sciences, Inc.
Hematology Laboratory
505 Coast Blvd. South
LaJolla, CA 92037
USA

Dr. U. G. Sauer
Akademie für Tierschutz
Spechtstrasse 1
D-85579 Neubiberg
Germany

T. H. Schilling
Institute of Tropical Medicine
University of Tübingen
Wilhelmstrasse 27
D-72074 Tübingen
Germany

Dr. H. Schulz-Key
Institute of Tropical Medicine
University of Tübingen
Wilhelmstrasse 27
D-72074 Tübingen
Germany

Dr. B. Sibanda
Advanced Tissue Sciences, Inc.
Hematology Laboratory
505 Coast Blvd. South
LaJolla, CA 92037
USA

Dr. J. A. Southee
Microbiologicals Ass. Int.
University of Stirling
Innovation Park
Stirling, Scotland FK9 4LA
UK

Prof. Dr. H. Spielmann
ZEBET
Robert von Ostertag Institut
des BGA
Postfach 480 447
D-12254 Berlin
Germany

Dr. H. M. Van Looy
OECD Environment Directorate
2 rue André Pascal
F-75775 Paris
France

Prof. Dr. L. F. M. van Zutphen
Dept. of Laboratory Animal Science
Faculty of Veterinary Medicine
Utrecht University
P.O. Box 80.166
3805 TD Utrecht
The Netherlands

Dr. A. Vedani
Swiss Institute for Alternatives
to Animal Testing (SIAT)
Biographics Laboratory
Aeschstrasse 14
CH-4107 Ettingen
Switzerland

A. Vollmer
Institute of Tropical Medicine
University of Tübingen
Wilhelmstrasse 27
D-72074 Tübingen
Germany

A. Welzel
Institute of Tropical Medicine
University of Tübingen
Wilhelmstrasse 27
D-72074 Tübingen
Germany

Contents

Preface   V

In memoriam   IX

Foreword   XI

List of contributors   XIII

1   Looking Back 33 Years to Russell and Burch: The Development of the
    Concept of the Three Rs (Alternatives)   1
    A. N. Rowan

2   The OECD and International Regulatory Acceptance of the Three Rs   13
    H. M. Van Looy, H. B. W. M. Koëter

3   The European Centre for the Validation of Alternative Methods
    (ECVAM)   21
    E. Marafante, M. Balls

4   A Timetable for Replacing, Reducing and Refining Animal Use with
    the Help of in Vitro Tests: The Limulus Amebocyte Lysate Test (LAL)
    as an Example   27
    O. Flint

5   The Fund for the Replacement of Animals in Medical Experiments
    (FRAME): 23 Years of Campaigning for the Three Rs   45
    M. Balls, J. H. Fentem

6   Animal Use and Alternatives: Developments in the Netherlands   57
    L. F. M. van Zutphen

7   The RIVM Center for Alternatives to Animal Testing and the Concept
    of the Three Rs in the Quality Control of Vaccines   67
    C. F. M. Hendriksen

8   ZEBET: Three Years of the National German Center for Documen-
    tation and Evaluation of Alternatives to Animal Experiments at the
    Federal Health Office (BGA) in Berlin   75
    H. Spielmann, B. Grune-Wolff, M. Liebsch

9   Reviewed Literature Databank for Alternatives to Animal Experiments
    – "Gelbe Liste"   85
    B. Rusche, U. G. Sauer

10   The SIAT Research, Teaching and Consulting Program in the Area of in Vitro Toxicology. Experimental Research, Screening and Validation 89
     C. A. Reinhardt

11   Computer-Aided Drug Design and the Three Rs   99
     A. Vedani

12   Computer-Aided Programs in Biomedical Education   107
     R. T. Fosse

13   Alternatives to Experiments with Animals in Medical Education: A TEMPUS Joint European Project   119
     M. Červinka, Z. Červinková, M. Balls, H. Spielmann

14   Replacement of Laboratory Animals in the Management of Blood-Sucking Arthropods   125
     A. E. Issmer, T. H. Schilling, A. Vollmer, J. Grunewald

15   Maintenance of Filarial Cycles in the Laboratory: Approaches to Replacing the Vertebrate Host   131
     J. Rapp, W. H. Hoffmann, L. Keller, A. Welzel, H. Schulz-Key

16   Improved Drug Metabolizing Capacity of Hepatocytes Co-Cultured with Epithelial Cells and Maintained in a Perifusion System   141
     R. Gebhardt

17   Characterization and Use of Long-Term Liver Cultures to Evaluate the Toxicity of Cyclophosphamide or Benzene to Bone Marrow Cultures
     147
     B. A. Naughton, B. Sibanda, J. San Román, G. K. Naughton

18   European Interlaboratory Evaluation of an in Vitro Ocular Irritation Model (Skin^{2TM} Model ZK1100) Using 18 Chemicals and Formulated Products   159
     P. W. Joller, A. Coquette, J. Noben, R. Pirovano, J. A. Southee, P. K. Logemann

19   Cellular Assays for Testing Peritoneal Dialysis Bags   165
     M. Dawson, Z. Jabar

20   The Position of the Authorities   173
     L. Pioda

Subject index   177

1 Looking Back 33 Years to Russell and Burch: The Development of the Concept of the Three Rs (Alternatives)

Andrew N. Rowan

Summary

The history of the alternatives concept, starting with the contribution by Russell and Burch, is outlined. Russell (a zoologist) and Burch (a microbiologist) were given the task of analyzing the ethical aspects of experimental techniques using animals by the British organization, the Universities Federation for Animal Welfare, in 1954. In 1959, they published a book which enunciated the principles of *Replacement*, *Reduction*, and *Refinement* (now known as the Three Rs or *alternatives*). Initially, their book was largely ignored but their ideas were gradually picked up by the animal protection community in the sixties and early seventies. In the eighties, spurred on by public pressure, the European biomedical research organizations and industry in Europe and America embraced the idea of alternatives. Concurrently, the demand for animals in research fell by up to 50%. Refinement, the often overlooked third R, is now also receiving much more attention.

Abbreviations. ATLA = Alternatives To Laboratory Animals; BGA = BundesGesundheits-Amt (Ministry of Health); BUAV = British Union for the Abolition of Vivisection; CAAT = Center for Alternatives to Animal Testing; CAM = ChorioAllantoic Membrane; ERGATT = European Research Group for Alternatives in Toxicity Testing; FRAME = Fund for the Replacement of Animals in Medical Experiments; HPLC = High Pressure Liquid Chromatography; IACUC = Institutional Animal Care and Use Committee; NAS = National Academy of Sciences (U. S. A.); NAVS = National AntiVivisection Society (U. K.); NIH = National Institutes of Health (U. S. A.); OECD = Organization for Economic Cooperation and Development; SSPV = Scottish Society for the Prevention of Vivisection (now Advocate for Animals); UFAW = Universities Federation for Animal Welfare; ZEBET = Zentralstelle zur Erfassung und Bewertung von Ersatz- und Ergänzungsmethoden zum Tierversuch.

1.1 Introduction

While most people cite Russell and Burch's (1959) book, *Principles of Humane Experimental Technique*, as the beginning of the concept of alternatives, there were earlier hints at the idea in discussions about appropriate use of animals in research. For example, Marshall Hall, a British experimental physiologist during the first half of the nineteenth century, proposed

Alternatives to Animal Testing. New Ways in the Biomedical Sciences, Trends and Progress.
Reinhardt, C. A. (ed.). 1994. © VCH, Weinheim.

five principles for animal experimentation that would eliminate unnecessary and repetitive procedures and would minimize suffering (Manuel, 1987). He also recommended the use of lower, less sentient animals and praised the findings of a colleague who demonstrated that an animal that had just been killed could be substituted for a living animal; thereby eliminating pain.

Fifty years after Hall set out these principles, a short-lived research trust (the Leigh Brown Trust) was established to promote and encourage scientific research without inflicting pain on experimental animals (French, 1975). Although the trust commissioned several publications, it never succeeded in developing a research program that convinced any significant proportion of the research community to adopt its principles. From 1900 to 1950, those who opposed the use of animals lost much of their political influence and were relegated to the fringes of political activity. As a result, not much attention was paid to the ethical questions posed by the use of animals in research.

After the Second World War, interest in the animal research issue began to grow again. In the United States, new animal protection groups were formed that began to criticize animal research practices and, in England, the Three Rs concept of alternatives began to emerge from the work of the Universities Federation for Animal Welfare (UFAW). In 1947, UFAW published a handbook on the care and management of laboratory animals (Worden, 1947), which was very well received. This gave UFAW the confidence, with the encouragement of some of their member scientists such as Sir Peter Medawar, to address the more contentious topic of experimental techniques (as opposed to animal care). Accordingly, in 1954, Major Hume (the founder of UFAW and its director at the time) sponsored a systematic examination of the progress of humane technique in the laboratory, employing Dr. William Russell (a young zoologist) and Mr. Rex Burch (a microbiologist) on the project (Hume, 1962b).

The origin of the *Three Rs* concept is not entirely clear. In a 1949 paper on the topic of befriending laboratory animals, Hume notes that in "the assay of therapeutic substances a choice of alternative techniques is often available" (Hume, 1962a). However, the context indicates that he was merely using the term *alternative* in its standard English sense and not as it is now interpreted by most of the animal protection movement and biomedical research organizations. Later, in a 1959 talk, Hume indicated that Russell was the originator of the Three Rs concept (Hume, 1962b).

The first recorded mention of the Three Rs was at a meeting on Humane Technique in the Laboratory, under the chairmanship of Sir Peter Medawar, organized by UFAW on May 7, 1957. Russell (1957) gave a presentation at this meeting in which he described the Three Rs. A brief proceedings (Anon., 1957) was published later that year by the Laboratory Animals Bureau of the Medical Research Council. Many of the arguments and ideas presented by Russell and the other speakers later appeared in *The Principles of Humane Experimental Technique* (Russell and Burch, 1959). This has now become the classic text on alternatives (and has recently been reprinted: Russell and Burch, 1992), but it apparently received little attention at the time despite its promotion by UFAW in England and the Animal Welfare Institute in the United States (see Table 1-1, which details the growing attention to Russell and Burch via citation analysis).

There are several examples of the lukewarm reaction to the book. In *Nature*, Weatherall (1959) comments that "it is useful to have a résumé of ways which have already been adopted to make experimentation as humane as possible. ... [but] It is not sufficiently informative to be used as guide either to details of experimental design or to the husbandry of experimental

Table 1-1. Citations to Russell and Burch from 1972 to 1991.

Period	Number of citations		Number of authors citing
	Per 4-year period	Cumulative	Cumulative
1972–1975	0	0	0
1976–1979	5	5	5
1980–1983	11	16	15
1984–1987	19	35	25
1988–1991	18	53	40

animals. Perhaps its chief purpose is to stimulate thought on both of these topics, and it is to be hoped it will succeed in doing so." The *Veterinary Record* reviewer (Anon., 1959) commented that the book contained an important message but found the philosophy "somewhat difficult reading" and hoped that the book would not be relegated "to the shelves merely for reference." *The Lancet* (Anon., 1960) also found the book difficult going, noting that "its purpose is admirable, and its matter unexceptionable" but "it is not easy reading." It is not clear whether the tepid reviewer reaction was the result of the book's arguments (a *Nature* review of a book that defended the use of animals (LaPage, 1960) was, by contrast, full of praise) or of a general lack of interest in the topic.

1.2   The 1960s

After the initial reviews in the scientific literature, the Russell and Burch book disappeared for almost ten years, although one began to see mention of the idea of alternatives from time to time. Geoffrey LaPage (1960), who described the contributions of animal research to medical advance, mentioned Russell and Burch and the concept of the Three Rs only once in a final chapter. He notes that distinguished scientists at a meeting organized by the Universities Federation for Animal Welfare

> ...discussed, among other things, how the numbers of laboratory animals used, and the numbers of experiments done on them, could be reduced, how their welfare could be improved, how the techniques used could be refined and how far, as Russell and Burch (1959) also discuss, animals could be replaced, for certain kinds of experiments at any rate. (p. 226)

In the U. S. A. in the early 1960s, there were several Congressional hearings on bills to regulate animal research. The printed record of the 1962 hearings is 375 pages long, but only one reference to Russell and Burch could be found and none at all to alternatives (U. S. Congress, 1962). The one reference to Russell and Burch came in testimony by Major Hume, the Director of UFAW, who had been flown over to the United States to testify that the Cruelty to Animals Act (1876) was well regarded by British scientists. In the same year, the Humane Society of the United States published a small booklet, *Animals in Research*, that reported the results of an analysis of the statistical approach used in published research papers by Westat Research Analysts (Anon., 1962). The analysts concluded that statistical design was usually inadequate and that savings in animal use of 25 % or more could have been effected without altering the validity of the results.

There were several other significant developments in the alternatives saga in the decade of the sixties. In 1962, the Lawson Tait Trust was established by the three leading U. K. antivivisection societies (BUAV, NAVS, and SSPV) to encourage and support researchers who were not using any animals in their research, and the Home Office set up a Committee of Inquiry into the workings of the 1876 Act, chaired by Sir Sidney Littlewood. The Littlewood Committee report was published in 1965. Significantly, it did address the question of alternatives, albeit only briefly. This indicated that the issue was beginning to be raised in public discourse. The Committee reported that it had

> ...repeatedly questioned scientific witnesses about the existence of alternative methods which would avoid the use of living animals. The replies have been unanimous in assuring us that such methods are actively sought and when found are readily adopted. ... Discoveries of adequate substitutes for animal tests have, however, so far been uncommon, and we have not been encouraged to believe that they are likely to be more frequent in the future. (Littlewood Committee, 1965, par. 71)

The Committee accepted these arguments and concluded that the demand for the use of animals in biomedical research was likely to increase in the coming years and that the discovery of substitutes for animal tests was not likely to affect the demand for animal experimentation.

The next recorded development was the establishment of the United Action for Animals in the United States in 1967 to promote alternatives and to focus on the principle of replacement. Its founder, Eleanor Seiling, spent many hours in the New York Public Library poring through scientific journals looking for examples of unnecessary animal research and of alternatives. However, she appears to have been a lone voice in the United States. Animal protection literature did not pay much attention to the idea of alternatives and it was virtually absent from the technical literature. According to an analysis by Phillips and Sechzer (1989), the term alternatives did not appear in the scientific literature on the animal research issue in the 1960s, although one 1966 paper did allude to the concept.

In 1969 in the U. K., FRAME (Fund for the Replacement of Animals in Medical Experiments) was established to promote the concept of alternatives among scientists, while the National Antivivisection Society set up the Lord Dowding Fund to support alternatives research. Both organizations were relatively well received by some popular science magazines (both the *New Scientist* and *World Medicine* praised the new, more scientific approach represented by the two organizations). Also in 1969, Sir Peter Medawar commented on the prospects for alternatives and predicted a decline in animal use.

> The use of animals in laboratories to enlarge our understanding of nature is part of a far wider exploratory process, and one cannot assay its value in isolation – as if it were an activity which, if prohibited, would deprive us only of the material benefits that grow directly out of its own use. Any such prohibition of learning or confinement of the understanding would have widespread and damaging consequences; but this does not imply that we are forevermore, and in increasing numbers, to enlist animals in the scientific service of man. I think that the use of experimental animals on the present scale is a

temporary episode in biological and medical history, and that its peak will be reached in ten years time, or perhaps even sooner. In the meantime, we must grapple with the paradox that nothing but research on animals will provide us with the knowledge that will make it possible for us, one day, to dispense with the use of them altogether. (Medawar, 1972, p. 86)

However, attitudes in the U. S. A. were more negative. A 1971 editorial in the *Journal of the American Medical Association* criticized FRAME in scathing terms (Anon., 1971), commenting that FRAME might be better named FRAUDS (Fund for the Replacement of Animals Used in the Discovery of Science).

1.3   The 1970s

In the 1970s, alternatives, or the Three Rs, became a central theme for the growing (in both size and political clout) animal protection movement (Rowan, 1989), and Russell and Burch began to be recognized as a seminal contribution to the animal research debate (see Table 1-1). It should be noted that the alternatives issue is the only new element in the argument about animal research. All the other arguments for and against the practice were exhaustively debated at the end of the nineteenth century (French, 1975; Turner, 1980).

Interest in alternatives began to grow dramatically in the 1970s among animal protection groups and among their public supporters. For example, the Humane Society of the United States established a committee of experts on alternatives in the early seventies. The establishment also began to be drawn into the debate, as indicated by some selected events (Table 1-2). The first major establishment initiative on alternatives came in 1971 when the Council of Europe passed Resolution 621. This proposed, among other things, the establishment of a documentation and information center on alternatives and tissue banks for research. Deliberations on Resolution 621 did not begin until the late seventies, and the final Council of Europe Convention that resulted dropped some of the specific recommendations

Table 1-2. Alternatives chronology, 1970–1979.

Year	Event
1971	Council of Europe Resolution 621 Ames Test
1972	Felix Wankel Prize for Animal Protection
1973	*ATLA Abstracts* founded (FRAME)
1975	Hybridoma technique developed (Köhler and Milstein, 1975) National Academy of Sciences Meeting (U. S. A.)
1977	Netherlands Animal Protection Law: Section on alternatives
1978	FRAME meeting at the Royal Society Smyth book on alternatives (from Research Defense Society)
1979	HR 4805 (U. S. A.): Research Modernization Act Sweden: established $90 000 of government funding for alternatives

on alternatives. Instead, the Convention reflected the broad concern over animal research and made some rather general recommendations on alternatives.

In Europe, a number of countries (e. g. the Netherlands and Sweden) had enacted animal research legislation by the end of the decade that included specific support for alternatives. For example, the Dutch Minister of Health confirmed his government's support for alternatives at the 1979 general meeting of the International Committee on Laboratory Animal Sciences in Utrecht. In Sweden, the government established an advisory Central Committee on Experimental Animals to develop and promote alternatives and allocated $90 000 annually for the support of research on alternatives (the first government funding for alternatives). The Federal Republic of Germany, Denmark, and Switzerland also passed regulations for laboratory animal protection which explicitly cover the development of alternatives. In the U. K., FRAME started *ATLA Abstracts* to identify articles in the published literature that focused on alternatives. While the journal had little impact when it was merely publishing abstracts, it started to include review articles in 1976 and then, early in the 1980s, dropped the abstracts altogether and adopted its current format. *ATLA* is now well enough established to be covered by the Science Citation Index.

In the U. S. A., interest in alternatives grew slowly. By the time the National Academy of Sciences organized a meeting on alternatives in 1975 (NAS, 1977), the term had entered the vocabulary of the animal movement on a large scale and had begun to find its way into the scientific literature (Phillips and Sechzer, 1989). Even so, the scientific community was not happy about the idea of alternatives and there was much criticism of the NAS for providing a platform for "anti-vivisectionists" by organizing the meeting. At the end of the 1970s, Eleanor Seiling of United Action for Animals managed to persuade a New York Congressman to introduce the Research Modernization Act. This act called on the National Institutes of Health (NIH) to reallocate 30–50 % of all money spent on animal research to alternatives. (Note: Seiling did not use the term *alternatives* to refer to the Three Rs, her "alternatives" referred only to Replacement.) The Research Modernization Act caught the imagination of the animal protection movement in spite of or, perhaps, because of its ambiguous language and lack of contact with political realities. This public pressure then forced Congress to start to pay attention to alternatives.

1.4   The 1980s

If the 1970s saw a gradual increase in interest in alternatives, the 1980s saw alternatives come of age, especially in Europe. It is not possible to produce a one-page chronology of significant events on alternatives for the decade, because so much has happened that one needs a single page to describe just a single year's events by the second half of the decade. Table 1-3 provides a listing of the most significant events from 1980 to 1985, but then government and private activities picked up dramatically.

In 1986, the Council of Environmental Ministers of the European Communities passed EEC Directive 86/609, which required member countries to develop enabling legislation promoting the Three Rs. The Animals (Scientific Procedures) Act 1986, replacing the 1876 Cruelty to Animals Act, was passed in the U. K. It required even greater attention to the issue of animal suffering (Refinement). In Germany, several government initiatives to validate alternative tests (ZEBET-BGA) were started. In the Netherlands, government officials

Table 1-3. Chronology 1980–1985.

1980	Spira Draize Campaign (U.S.A.)
1981	Johns Hopkins University Center for Alternatives to Animal Testing (U.S.A.)
	Swiss legislation requires consideration of alternatives
	Zbinden and Flury-Roversi paper criticizing the classical LD_{50}
1982	Colgate Palmolive provides $300000 to investigate CAM system (U.S.A.)
1983	Switzerland provides SFr 2 million over 2 years for alternatives research
1984	FRAME (U.K.) receives £160000 from Home Office. First U.K. government funding for alternatives research
1985	U.S.A.: Health Research Extension Act is passed requiring NIH to develop a plan for alternatives
	U.S.A.: Animal Welfare Act Amendments are passed that require greater attention to alternatives in research that causes pain and distress
	Index Medicus adds a subject heading: Alternatives to Animal Testing
	European Research Group for Alternatives in Toxicity Testing (ERGATT) is formed

collected data on the extent of the suffering experienced by laboratory animals, and the OECD, driven by representatives from European countries, began to address the Three Rs in their guidelines for toxicity testing.

Worldwide, probably the most significant event in the eighties was the launching of campaigns in many of the developed countries against animal testing of cosmetics, toiletries, and household products. These campaigns built on the efforts and publications during the late seventies by such organizations as FRAME in the U.K. that laid out the scientific challenges to the routine use of animals in toxicity testing (Balls *et al.*, 1983; Zbinden and Flury-Roversi, 1981). The main actor in the animal protection campaigns was a labor and civil rights activist named Henry Spira who turned his attention to animals after reading an article by the Australian philosopher, Peter Singer (1973). He made contacts with activists in England (such as Jean Pink of Animal Aid, who had been targeting cosmetics testing since 1977), continental Europe and Australia and helped to focus and coordinate protests against the eye irritancy testing (the Draize test) of cosmetics worldwide.

In the U.S.A., Spira's Draize test campaign built a coalition of 400 animal protection organizations which targeted use of the Draize eye test by cosmetic companies and Revlon in particular. Within 12 months, the coalition's activities resulted in over $1.75 million of funding for alternatives research. The Rockefeller University received $750000 from Revlon to establish a laboratory for in vitro toxicological assay development, and the Johns Hopkins University Center for Alternatives to Animal Testing (CAAT) was established with $1 million from the Cosmetic, Toiletry, and Fragrance Association, Inc. Avon Products, Inc., Bristol-Myers Squibb, and other companies provided the bulk of the funds for CAAT and also provided funds for FRAME programs in the U.K.

The effectiveness of Spira's campaign was based on several factors. First, he engaged in extensive preliminary planning and preparation. For example, Spira acquired numerous copies of the government Draize test training film and slides (showing inflamed and damaged rabbit eyes) *before* the campaign started. By late 1980, these materials were no longer being handed out free to anyone who asked. Second, he did not shy away from the hard-nosed street politics he had learned in the labor and civil rights campaigns and he made skillful use of demonstrations and the media. Third, he was always willing to negotiate with the opposition and he avoided personal attacks and insults. This earned him the respect of his opponents. Fourth, he engaged in a constant search for solutions in which everybody could feel they had won something. Also, he did not boast to the media about victories over corporate targets. When Revlon finally negotiated a settlement with Spira that set up the Rockefeller alternatives research program, Spira not only stopped his campaign, but he also praised Revlon for their innovative initiative and invited other cosmetic companies to take similarly progressive steps.

The impact of the Draize campaign on the question of alternatives in toxicity testing was enormous. From 1981 to 1991, there was a tremendous shift in attitude toward alternatives in toxicity testing within industry. Corporate toxicologists who went along with the initial grants for alternatives research in 1980 and 1981 because they felt such actions were necessary for public relations reasons, became excited by the technical and scientific challenge of alternatives by the end of the decade. Colgate-Palmolive began to fund research into the CAM test in 1982 (to the amount of $300 000) and within three years had set up an alternatives program in their in-house laboratories. Procter and Gamble and Bristol-Myers Squibb made the search for alternatives part of their corporate culture and currently provide millions of dollars annually for intramural and extramural alternatives programs. Industrial In Vitro Toxicology associations have been started in both Europe and the United States and several toxicology journals specializing in in vitro approaches were established in the late 1980s.

Despite all the interest, however, people are still cautious about relying too heavily on the new in vitro techniques. Toxicological risk evaluation is a very difficult art, and the move from laboratory prototype alternatives to their use as replacements for whole animals has not occurred (except in a few, well-defined instances). However, there is now widespread consensus that toxicology testing needs to move in a different direction. Thus, at the first symposium (in 1982) of the Johns Hopkins Center for Alternatives to Animal Testing, the participants mostly wondered *if* an alternative to the Draize could be found (Goldberg, 1983) but, within five years, participants at CAAT symposia were discussing *when* an alternative would be available.

While similar developments are evident in Europe, there is a large segment of scientists outside industry that have yet to embrace the concept of alternatives in America. In fact, important research institutions such as the NIH avoid any use of the term alternatives whenever possible. For example, the Health Research Extension Act of 1985 required NIH to establish an alternatives program, which ended up with the awkward title Biomedical Models and Materials Resources. A few years later, a Public Health Service draft document on animal welfare commented that "efforts have led to the discovery of research methods that are useful as 'adjuncts' to animal research, in that they complement animal models but rarely replace them. Thus, these adjuncts are not true 'alternatives' – even the use of this latter term can be misleading" (U. S. Public Health Service, 1989). Other biomedical research advocates have argued that use of the term alternatives implies that one needs to apologize for using animals in research and that this gives the public the wrong impression (Goodwin, 1992). Biomedical research in the U. S. is, thus, decidedly schizophrenic on the subject of alternatives. There is a small but growing industry of in vitro toxicology companies to service corporate needs, but academic research tries to deny any validity to the alternatives concept.

Despite such pockets of resistance, technical developments throughout the developed world have led to substantial changes in animal use. Most countries that keep records on animal research use report a fall in laboratory animal numbers during the 1980s, in some cases, a dramatic fall. The statistics from the United Kingdom show a decline in annual animal use from around 5.5 million in 1976 to a little over 3 million in 1987 (Anon., 1990). Sir Peter Medawar, who, in 1969, predicted that such a decline would begin in 1979 or even earlier (Medawar, 1972), was obviously more far-sighted than the Littlewood Committee who, in 1965, reported that animal use would not be influenced by the development of new (alternative) technology.

However, one immediate question is how much of the decline in research animal use in the U.K. and in other countries can be attributed primarily to the development and use of alternative methods? The available data is not adequate to provide an unequivocal answer. While other factors such as the costs of research animals and the increased sensitivity and specificity of new techniques have no doubt been important, it is also likely that pressure from animal groups calling for the development and use of *alternative* techniques has played a significant role in reducing animal use.

Technical developments over the past 30 years have, for example, reduced the demand for animals in the production and testing of polio vaccine and insulin (Hendriksen, 1988; Trethewey, 1989). Hendriksen describes how the number of monkeys used in the production and testing of polio vaccine in the Netherlands was reduced from 4570 in 1965 to 30 in 1984 by a series of technical improvements, although the actual amount of polio vaccine produced was about the same in the two years. The technical improvements included in situ trypsinization of monkey kidneys to improve the yield of cells from each kidney, introduction of microcarrier technology to increase polio virus yield from cell culture, and the use of subcultured (tertiary cells) rather than primary cells as virus substrates.

Trethewey describes a similar process in insulin testing that reduced the demand for mice by 95 % between 1970 and 1986. The major technical advance was the introduction of a mouse blood glucose test in place of the mouse convulsion test. This relatively non-stressful assay permitted the re-use of the same mouse for more than one assay, leading to a further reduction in the number of animals required. HPLC techniques have been developed and introduced, and it is now possible to standardize insulin preparations using only a handful of mice to ensure that each batch is biologically active. A life-time supply of insulin for one diabetic now requires testing on the equivalent of only a single mouse, and it is possible that mice will be eliminated altogether as further technical advances are made.

Refinements in toxicity testing and the standardization of therapeutics have reduced the demand for animals in some tests. However, the most significant reductions have come in the search for new drugs. As pharmaceutical companies have switched from animal to in vitro screens for agents with potential therapeutic activity, they have recorded dramatic decreases in animal use. Hoffman-La Roche, for example, reduced its annual animal use from 1 million to about 300 000 without changing the number of new drug entities under investigation (Anon., 1990). A relatively recent switch by the National Cancer Institute from a mouse screen for potential anti-cancer agents to human cancer cell culture screens has resulted in a saving of several million mice per year (Rowan and Andrutis, 1990).

In the last eight years, public and legislative support for alternatives has continued to grow. New legislation in Europe emphasizes the need to consider alternatives, while Institutional Animal Care and Use Committees (IACUCs) in the U.S.A. are being pressured by Animal Welfare Act inspectors to demand that investigators provide a written statement of what they have done to look for alternative methods. While animal numbers continue to decline (although the numbers went up in the U. K. in 1991 for the first time in over a decade), more attention is now being paid to the neglected R – Refinement. In the U. K., the debate over and the passage of the 1986 Animals (Scientific Procedures) Act focused more attention on animal distress and has led to a virtual doubling (from 21 % to 36 % of all procedures) in the rate of anesthetic use in animal research in six years (Anon., 1990). In the U. S. A., protocol review by IACUCs tends to focus on minimizing pain and distress in the animals, and this has led to increased attention to the alleviation of animal distress by a variety of public and private organizations.

1.5   Conclusion

The program that Major Hume set in motion in 1954 has born significant fruit in the following 40 years. Although he would no doubt be surprised at the scope and potential of biomedical science today, Major Hume would be pleased at the recognition accorded to Russell and Burch (1959). In 1959, he spoke as follows to an Animal Care Panel meeting in Washington, DC:

> A more recent event has been the publication of a remarkable book by Russell and Burch entitled *The Principles of Humane Experimental Technique*. This deserves to become a classic for all time, and we have great hopes that it will inaugurate a new field of systematic study. We hope that others will follow up the lead it has given, and that a generalized study of humane technique, as a systematic component of the methodology of research, will come to be considered essential to the training of a biologist. (Hume, 1962b)

References

Anonymous (1957) *Laboratory Animals Bureau Collected Papers,* Vol. 6. Laboratory Animals Bureau, Hampstead, London.

Anonymous (1959) [Review of *The Principles of Humane Experimental Technique*]. *Veterinary Record* **71,** 650.

Anonymous (1960) [Review of *The Principles of Humane Experimental Technique*]. *The Lancet* **i, 34.**

Anonymous (1962) *Animals in Research.* Humane Society of the United States, Washington, DC.

Anonymous (1971) Antivisection rides again. *JAMA* **217,** 70.

Anonymous (1990) Statistics on the three R's. *The Alternatives Report* **2,** 1–15.

Balls M., Riddell R.J. and Worden A.N. (Editors) (1983) *Animals and Alternatives in Toxicity Testing.* Academic Press, London.

French R.D. (1975) *Antivivisection and Medical Science in Victorian Society.* Princeton University Press, Princeton, NJ.

Goldberg A.M. (Editor) (1983) *Product Safety Evaluation, Vol. 1. Alternative Methods in Toxicology.* Mary Ann Liebert Inc., New York.

Goodwin F.K. (1992) Animal research, animal rights and public health. *Conquest, The Journal of the Research Defence Society* **181,** 1–10.

Hendriksen C.F.M. (1988) *Laboratory Animals in Vaccine Production and Control.* Kluwer Academic Publishers, Dordrecht.

Hume C. W. (1962a) How to befriend laboratory animals. In *Man and Beast.* C. W. Hume. pp. 115–137. Universities Federation for Animal Welfare, Potters Bar, Herts, UK.

Hume, C.W. (1962b) The vivisection controversy in Britain. In *Man and Beast.* C.W. Hume. pp. 57–70. Universities Federation for Animal Welfare, Potters Bar, Herts, UK.

Köhler G. and Milstein C. (1975) Continuous culture of fused cells secreting anitbody of predefined specificity. *Nature* **256**, 495–497.

LaPage, G. (1960) *Achievement: Some Contributions of Animal Experiment to the Conquest of Disease.* W. Heffer & Sons, Cambridge, UK.

Littlewood Committee (1965) *Report of the Departmental Committee on Experiements in Animals.* Her Majesty's Stationery Office, London.

Manuel D. (1987) Marshall Hall (1770–1857): Vivisection and the development of experimental physiology. In *Vivisection in Historical Perspective.* Edited by N.A. Rupke. pp. 87–104. Croom Helm, London.

Medawar P.B. (1972) *The Hope of Progress.* Methuen, London.

National Academy of Sciences (NAS) (1977) *The Future of Animals, Cells, Models and Systems in Research, Development, Education and Testing.* National Academy of Sciences, Washington, DC.

Phillips M.T. and Sechzer J.A. (1989) *Animal Research and Ethical Conflict: An Analysis of the Scientific Literature, 1966–1986.* Springer Verlag, Berlin.

Rowan A.N. (1989) The development of the animal protection movement. *Journal of NIH Research* **1**, 97–100.

Rowan A.N. and Andrutis K.A. (1990) NCI's developmental therapeutics program. *The Alternatives Report* **2**, 1, 3.

Russell W.M.S. (1957) The increase of humanity in experimentation: replacement, reduction and refinement. *Laboratory Animals Bureau, Collected Papers* **6**, 23–26.

Russell W.M.S. and Burch R.L. (1959) *The Principles of Humane Experimental Technique.* Methuen, London.

Russell W.M.S. and Burch R.L. (1992) *The Principles of Humane Experimental Technique.* Reprinted by Universities Federation for Animal Welfare, Potters Bar, Herts., U.K.

Singer, P. (1973) [Review of *Animals, Men and Morals*]. *The New York Review of Books.* April 5, pp. 17–21.

Trethewey J. (1989) The development of insulin assays without the use of animals. In *In Vitro Toxicology: New Directions, Vol. 7. Alternative Methods in Toxicology.* Edited by A.M. Goldberg. pp. 113–122. Mary Ann Liebert Inc., New York.

Turner J. (1980) *Reckoning with the Beast: Animals, Pain and Humanity in the Victorian Mind.* Johns Hopkins University Press, Baltimore, MD.

U.S. Congress (1962) *Hearings before a Subcommittee of the Committee on Interstate and Foreign Commerce; House of Representatives, 87th Congress on H.R. 1937 and H.R. 3556, September 28 and 29.* U.S. Government Printing Office, Washington, DC.

U.S. Public Health Service (1989) *Final Report of the Public Health Service Animal Welfare Working Group, Phase I.* Department of Health and Human Services, Washington, DC.

Weatherall M. (1959) [Review of *The Principles of Humane Experimental Technique*]. *Nature* **184**, 1675–1676.

Worden A.N. (Editor) (1947) *The UFAW Handbook on the Care and Management of Laboratory Animals.* Bailliere, Tindall and Cox, London.

Zbinden G. and Flury-Roversi M. (1981) Significance of the LD50 test for the toxicological evaluation of chemical substances. *Archives of Toxicology* **47**, 77–99.

2 The OECD and International Regulatory Acceptance of the Three Rs

Hugo M. Van Looy and Herman B. W. M. Koëter

Summary

The work of the Organisation for Economic Cooperation and Development (OECD) has been pivotal in reaching a consensus on methods of testing that can be used to fulfill national regulatory requirements and, at the same time, to develop data that are acceptable in other countries. Within the program of the OECD, utmost attention is given to incorporating Three Rs improvements, whenever possible and practicable. Today, and for the purpose of regulatory testing, it seems that in vitro alternatives have the limited role of screening chemicals, i.e. identifying those for which full in vivo testing would be a useless and wasteful exercise. It is recognized that the scientific validation of promising in vitro methods is the safest route towards regulatory acceptance. But it is also recognized that this route is extremely resource intensive. An alternative route, that of confidence building, is suggested in this paper.

2.1 Introduction

This contribution from the Secretariat of OECD on the acceptance of Three Rs data for regulatory purposes documents the key position the OECD has taken in establishing international consensus on methods that can be used in the fulfilment of regulatory requirements of chemicals control. Many scientists may be little aware of the importance of this consensus, of how it is achieved, and what its implications are. In the first section, it will therefore briefly be explained a) why and how the Organisation became involved in methods for chemicals safety testing, b) how OECD guidelines for testing are developed and adopted, and c) what the scope of these guidelines is and where they are applied.

In 1982 a clear message was delivered by ministers of the OECD member countries urging the bodies of the Organisation involved in the program on test methods to make every effort possible to discover, develop, and validate alternative testing systems. In the second section it will be explained how this instruction has been carried out, what the Three Rs improvements have been, and what the future holds.

In the third section, some of the roadblocks to acceptance of alternative tests by authorities are discussed, whereby a distinction between reduction and refinement on the one hand and truly alternative in vitro systems on the other imposes itself. Issues of primary impor-

Alternatives to Animal Testing. New Ways in the Biomedical Sciences, Trends and Progress.
Reinhardt, C. A. (ed.). 1994. © VCH, Weinheim.

tance are a) the scientific justification of new methods, b) the reliability of the data obtained, and c) the complexity of validation.

The conclusions will focus primarily on what appears to be achievable today with respect to the regulatory use of in vitro methods. Currently, the role of in vitro methods within regulatory schemes of testing is mainly that of screening: exempting substances that gave a positive result in in vitro assays from full in vivo testing.

2.2   The OECD and methods for chemicals safety testing

In the seventies, several countries enacted, or were preparing, laws which imposed on chemical companies the detailed testing of new chemicals as part of notification procedures (the 1969 Swiss Law on Trade in Toxic Substances, the 1973 Japanese Chemical Substances Control Law, the 1976 U. S. Toxic Substances Control Act and the EC 6th Amendment of 1979). There was a real danger that, unless an international agreement on methods for testing was reached, data could be rejected on the basis that an inappropriate test had been used. Non-tariff trade barriers would result, and, in response to this threat, the OECD Chemicals Group launched the Chemicals Testing Program. Its objective was to prepare "state-of-the-art" reports on the best methods available for generating data useful for the purpose of hazard assessment. The program was met by great enthusiasm in the member countries and received great support from three sectors: government, industry, and academia. Five groups of experts (physical-chemical properties, ecotoxicological effects, degradation-accumulation, short-term health effects, and long-term health effects) held several meetings which were hosted by lead countries in the period 1978–1980. As the work progressed, a breakthrough was achieved with the idea of an official stamp for methods around which strong international consensus was reached. The term *OECD Guideline for Testing of Chemicals* was coined, and 51 guidelines were officially adopted by the Council of OECD in 1981 (OECD, 1981a).

2.3   The actual process of OECD test guidelines development

After 1981 the development of test guidelines continued. New guidelines were added and several existing guidelines were modified (updated). The way in which guidelines were processed from the proposal stage to the final official adoption changed somewhat over the years. The changes did not affect the underlying basic principle of consensus amongst the member countries, which is common to all OECD activities. The various steps of the current process are given in Figure 2-1 (Koëter, 1993). Some particularly important features of this scheme deserve attention.

In each member country a person is responsible for coordinating nationally the OECD activity on test guidelines. In general, these national coordinators are officials from a government department, agency, or institute in charge of environmental protection, who work in close collaboration with their counterparts in the public health sector. The national coordinators maintain an efficient network for consulting with national experts, who should represent as broadly as possible the country's expertise in the different areas of test methodology. A national coordinator, having established a good consensus amongst his (her) specialized national experts on a proposal for a new method or revised OECD guideline, submits the pro-

OECD TEST GUIDELINE DEVELOPMENT FLOW DIAGRAM

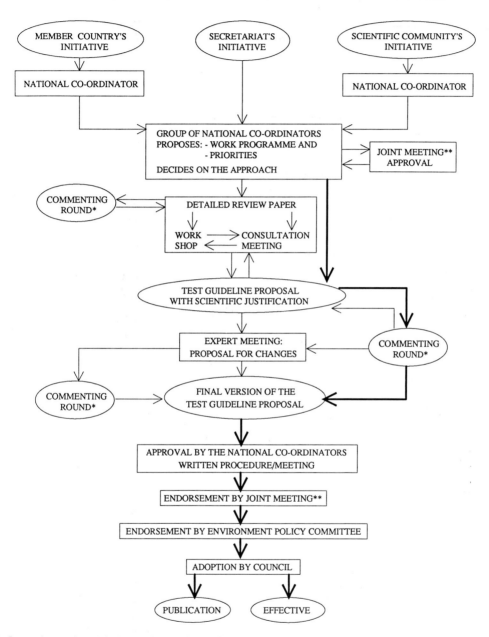

*   Commenting rounds would include Member countries, BIAC, and scientific societies, as appropriate.
** Joint Meeting of the Chemicals Group and Management Committee of the Special Programme on the Control of Chemicals.

⟶   = fast track procedure.

Figure 2-1. Diagram of the process of OECD test guideline development (Koëter, 1993).

posal to the Secretariat of the Organisation. The proposal is circulated to all other national coordinators who, after consulting their experts, emit national comments and views on the proposal. These are compiled by the Secretariat. In general, the compilation is submitted to the annual meeting of the national coordinators where a decision is taken on whether or not to do further work on the proposal.

The further work will inevitably be done by a group of experts whose task is to develop a draft guideline. On this draft guideline agreement is sought from the assembly of national coordinators and, after that, from the Chemicals Group. When this is achieved, the draft guideline is submitted to the Council for adoption.

There are alternatives to this process, and a major one derives from a conclusion reached by the Chemicals Group when it met at high level in 1987. That conclusion asked for a periodical revision of the OECD guidelines. To achieve this, first a review paper is written, covering a group of tests addressing similar endpoints, e. g. terrestrial ecotoxicity, biodegradation, skin irritation, mutagenicity, etc. The next step consists in the development of a suitable method to fill a gap identified in the review, or of a proposal for updating an existing guideline needing amendment. The proposals are then processed through commenting rounds and meetings of experts, as described in the previous paragraph.

2.4   The scope and application of OECD test guidelines

The *OECD Guidelines for Testing of Chemicals* are an inherent part of the Council Act C(81)30 (OECD, 1981b), by which the Council decided that "data generated in the testing of chemicals in an OECD Member country in accordance with the OECD Test Guidelines and OECD Principles of Good Laboratory Practice shall be accepted in other Member countries for purposes of assessment and other uses relating to the protection of man and the environment." Because council decisions are binding for the 24 member countries, it becomes immediately clear that a prerequisite for the international regulatory acceptance of any method, including Three Rs alternative methods, consists in getting the OECD guideline stamp.

The scope of application of the OECD test guidelines can be analyzed in relation to the meaning given to the word *chemicals*. In the council decision *chemicals* is not qualified. Although the origin of the OECD test guidelines goes back in reality to the harmonization of tests to be used in the notification of new chemicals, they are today applied in the regulatory testing of probably all categories of chemicals including pesticides, pharmaceuticals, and food additives. Although they do not cover all requirements, like those deriving from specific end-uses and particular exposure situations, being assembled in a unique compendium of internationally recognized methods, they are very widely applied.

2.5   Three Rs improvements in OECD test guidelines

The experts who developed the first guidelines on health effects during 1979/80 gave importance to considerations of animal welfare, as can be judged from the following quote from their summary report: "With the objective of an efficient approach to testing chemicals there is no point in having more groups or more animals per group than are strictly necessary to attain the end-point of the reliable detection of toxic effects" (OECD, 1981a). This consideration was reflected in several early health effects guidelines where the numbers of animals recommended were lower than in the methods which were then commonly practiced. The experts also introduced the concept of limit tests. If a test at one predetermined high dose produced no test substance related effects, a full study using several dose levels was considered unnecessary. In 1982, a high level meeting of the Chemicals Group adopted the following statement:

> The welfare of laboratory animals is important. It will continue to be an important factor influencing the work in the OECD Chemicals Program. The progress in OECD on the harmonization of chemicals control, in particular the agreement on mutual acceptance of data, by reducing duplicative testing, will do much to reduce the number of animals used in testing. Such testing cannot be eliminated at present, but every effort should be made to discover, develop and validate alternative testing systems.

In 1986, experts were convened to a meeting in Paris to discuss improvements to the guidelines on acute oral and dermal toxicity and eye irritation. At the meeting, consideration was given to the British Toxicology Society fixed dose procedure, the German tox class method, the up-and-down procedure, and the low volume eye irritation test. Sufficient general agreement on the applicability of any of these tests in the regulatory context was not reached. The meeting, however, made the following amendments (which were adopted in 1987) to the three existing guidelines:

Guidelines 401 (acute oral) and 402 (acute dermal):
– one sex tested;
– limit dose lowered to 2000 mg/kg;
– animals showing severe and enduring signs of distress and pain may need to be killed.

Guideline 405 (acute eye irritation/corrosion):
– if results from *well-validated* alternative tests show severe effects, further testing is not recommended;
– a tiered approach: start with one animal;
– a reduced number of animals for studying the rinsing effect.

Following an international validation study, adoption of the *fixed dose method* took place in 1992. It became *Guideline 420*.

During 1990, detailed review papers from the European Chemical Industry Ecology and Toxicology Centre (ECETOC) and the OECD Secretariat on skin irritation and sensitization became available (ECETOC, 1988, 1990a, 1990b). In the review papers, extensive consideration was given to Three Rs alternatives (Frazier, 1990). In May 1991, experts were convened in Paris to discuss the updating of the skin irritation/corrosion and the sensitization guidelines and also an area not yet covered by OECD guidelines, phototoxicity. Whereas work is being continued on the last subject mentioned, the meeting agreed on substantial Three Rs improvements (adopted in 1992) to the existing guidelines as follows:

Guideline 404 (acute dermal irritation/corrosion):
– a waiver for a full in vivo test on the basis of a positive result in an in vitro test (remark: no mention of *well validated* or specific tests);

– if an in vitro test is performed before the in vivo test, details of the in vitro test must be given in the test report together with the results obtained;
– tiered approach: start with one animal.

Guideline 406 (skin sensitization):
– the number of recommended methods is reduced from 7 to 2;
– reduction in the number of animals;
– a waiver for performing the recommended tests if a positive result is obtained in 1 of 2 recommended less invasive in vivo procedures (Mouse Ear Sensitization Test (MEST) and Local Lymph Node Assay (LLNA));
– results of these screening assays must be reported, if performed.

2.6   Acceptance of alternative tests for regulatory purposes

So far, most discussions on the acceptability of data from alternative tests have, probably rightly, given much importance to the scientific validation of the methods (Balls *et al.*, 1990b; van den Heuvel and Fielder, 1990). It is generally recognized that the traditional in vivo procedures were accepted without validation. The confidence in these methods rests on the widely held opinion that data obtained in whole animal models can be reliably extrapolated to humans. This confidence, with few exceptions, has gradually been strengthened by the experience gained. Acceptance of *Reduction* and *Refinement* improvements of the traditional methods has also been possible without validation. The fixed dose method went through validation before being accepted because, in this case, it was to be shown that the data allowed the correct entering of chemicals in existing LD_{50}-based classes of toxicity. Extensive validation is therefore rather typical of certain in vitro and ex vivo *Replacement* alternatives, e. g. when the new test is a clear-cut alternative to an existing test.

2.7   Conclusive validation and a side route to acceptance

Validation is very difficult for many reasons, which need not be elaborated for the purpose of this paper. The process that leads to it is extremely resource intensive and time consuming. Both aspects, the difficulty and the magnitude of the effort, were analyzed recently by Koëter (1993). The scientific approach toward acceptance through validation studies, regardless of how difficult and complex these may be (Balls *et al.*, 1990a; Frazier, 1990), remains an aim needing to be pursued. The validation of alternative methods shown to have a mechanistic similarity to the toxic effect addressed is more likely to be conclusive if the mechanism of the effect is understood. However, the evaluation of a systemic effect on the basis of data from alternative tests (by necessity a battery of them), represents a difficulty of higher order.

Given the difficulty of the systematic scientific approach to regulatory acceptance, a more pragmatic approach toward confidence building can be considered. Many alternative tests have been and are being developed, and it is difficult to decide which are the more powerful and promising ones. What is needed is a gradual development of a database linking alternative data with data from in vivo studies for a specific compound. This can be achieved in regulatory toxicity testing (perhaps for certain endpoints), and the modifications included in the updated OECD guidelines on skin irritation and sensitization, encouraging the submission of data from alternative tests in the report of the full study, are a first step in this direction. As the database develops, confidence in alternative methods that perform well will increase. A major advantage of this database would be that it would contain negative results of in vitro studies, which otherwise would never show up. This approach, in order to be successful, would need a concerted view of the scientific community as to what methods show the greatest promise.

2.8   Conclusions

We do agree with van den Heuvel and Fielder (1990) that "the major regulatory role of *in vitro* studies will, for some time yet, be in providing effective screening for specific local effects" and also that "the results from *in vitro* studies are becoming increasingly important to regulatory authorities by enabling the real need for animal studies to be evaluated." A very important application of in vitro tests is the direct use of positive results in a decision on classification and labeling without confirming the results in an animal test.

As far as the future is concerned, scientific justification, preferably supported by validation studies, will provide the means for identifying, and accepting for regulatory purposes, reliable alternative tests. The more conclusive the evidence that the alternative is mechanistically related to the toxic effect, the easier acceptance will be.

In the meantime, a pragmatic route to confidence building, by providing authorities in parallel with in vitro and in vivo data, is open. A condition for success along this route would be for the scientific community to reach an agreement on the most promising methods.

References

Balls M., Blaauboer B., Brusick D., Frazier J., Lamb D., Pemberton M., Reinhardt C., Roberfroid M., Rosenkranz H., Schmid B., Spielmann H., Stammati A.-L. and Walum E. (1990a) Report and recommendations of the CAAT/ERGATT workshop on the validation of toxicity test procedures. *ATLA* **18**, 313–337.

Balls M., Botham P., Cordier A., Fumero S., Kayser D., Koëter H., Koundakjian P., Lindquist N. G., Meyer O., Pioda L., Reinhardt C., Rozemond H., Smyrniotis T., Spielmann H., Van Looy H., van der Venne M.-T. and Walum E. (1990b) Report and recommendations of an international workshop on promotion of the regulatory acceptance of validated non-animal toxicity testing procedures. *ATLA* **18**, 339–344.

European Chemical Industry Ecology and Toxicology Centre (1988) *Eye Irritation Testing* (ECOTOC Monograph No. 11). ECETOC, Brussels.

European Chemical Industry Ecology and Toxicology Centre (1990a) *Skin Irritation* (ECOTOC Monograph No. 15). ECETOC, Brussels.

European Chemical Industry Ecology and Toxicology Centre (1990b) *Skin Sensitisation Testing* (ECOTOC Monograph No. 14). ECETOC, Brussels.

Frazier J. (1990) *Scientific Criteria for Validation of in vitro Toxicity Tests* (Environment Monographs No. 36). OECD Publications Office, Paris.

Koëter H. B. W. M. (1993) Test guideline development and animal welfare: Regulatory acceptance of *in vitro* studies. *Reproductive Toxicology 7* (Suppl.), 117–123.

Organisation for Economic Cooperation and Development. (1981a) *OECD Guidelines for Testing of Chemicals.* OECD Publications Office, Paris.

Organisation for Economic Cooperation and Development. (1981b) *Decision of the Council of 12th May 1981 Concerning the Mutual Acceptance of Data in the Assessment of Chemicals* (C(81)30(Final)). OECD Publications Office, Paris.

van den Heuvel M. J. and Fielder R. J. (1990) Acceptance of *in vitro* testing by regulatory authorities. *Toxicology in Vitro* **4**, 675–679.

3 The European Centre for the Validation of Alternative Methods (ECVAM)

Erminio Marafante and Michael Balls

Summary

At the end of 1991, the Commission of the European Communities informed the Council of Ministers and the European Parliament of its decision to set up a European Centre for the Validation of Alternative Methods (ECVAM), in line with its responsibilities under Directive 86/609/EEC. The main goal of ECVAM is to coordinate, at the European level, activities designed to promote the scientific and regulatory acceptance of alternative methods which are of importance to the biosciences and which reduce, refine or replace the use of laboratory animals. ECVAM is assisted by a Scientific Advisory Committee representative of all parties concerned with the validation of alternative methods, namely the Member States, and European industries, animal welfare organizations and academia. ECVAM is currently establishing information services and a series of workshops, task forces and symposia. It supports interlaboratory pre-validation and formal validation studies, and will itself also be practically involved in the development and validation of non-animal tests and testing strategies.

3.1 Foundation

In November 1986, the Council of the European Communities adopted Directive 86/609/EEC on the approximation of the laws, regulations, and administrative provisions of the Member States regarding the protection of animals used for experimental and other scientific purposes (EEC, 1986). Article 23 of this directive calls on the Commission and Member States to encourage the development and validation of alternative techniques that could provide the same level of information as those used at the time, but would involve fewer animals or entail less painful procedures.

The European Parliament subsequently called on the Commission to provide a mechanism for the validation of alternative testing methods, including, where necessary, the provision of financial support to the participating laboratories.

However, a Commission report to the Council later stated that "the Commission recognises that a critical stage in the development of an alternative method is the transition from that of a potentially useful procedure to that of a method accepted as part of a regulatory testing system." The Commission therefore declared its intention to provide a framework for the evaluation (validation) of alternative test procedures by establishing an appropriate European

Alternatives to Animal Testing. New Ways in the Biomedical Sciences, Trends and Progress.
Reinhardt, C. A. (ed.). 1994. © VCH, Weinheim.

body for coordinating the validation of alternative methods, i. e. a European center to cater to the needs identified in this area by the Council, the European Parliament and the Commission.

After assessing all possible options, the Commission decided to set up the center within the Joint Research Centre's Environment Institute at Ispra, Italy. This decision was taken because the center would be part of the JRC at Ispra and therefore in an environment that is neutral, multilingual, and has long been active in international scientific collaboration. This would enable it:

– to use the technical infrastructure of the JRC, which already had toxicological laboratories with facilities for conducting experiments in vitro and at the molecular level;
– to benefit from the multidisciplinary scientific support of the JRC, which has lengthy experience in database management and in the validation of protocols and methods of analysis in various fields; and
– to help to expand the JRC's role in prenormative research.

Clearly, however, a center of this kind would be unable to perform its tasks to the full, unless it could rely on the cooperation and expertise of all parties concerned, namely, the Member States, industrial companies, the academic world, and animal welfare organizations. It was therefore proposed that a Scientific Advisory Committee be set up, on which all those parties and the Commission would be represented, and which would have the task of advising the center and helping it to set priorities when drawing up its annual work program.

3.2   Establishment and functions

In practical terms, this means that a *special administrative unit*, to be known as the European Centre for the Validation of Alternative Methods (ECVAM), is being set up within the Environment Institute of the JRC. Its primary task will be to coordinate the validation of alternative test methods at the European Community level. This will involve the specification of test protocols, the organization of ring-test exercises, the choice of chemicals to be used in these tests, and the analysis and evaluation of the results, etc. In addition to this main activity, the Centre will also have the following functions:

– to act as a focal point for the exchange of information on the development of alternative methods;
– to set up, maintain and manage a database on alternative procedures, with associated user services (help line, advice service, etc.); and
– to promote dialog among legislators, industrial companies, biomedical scientists, consumer organizations, and animal welfare groups, with a view to the development, validation, and international recognition of non-animal test methods.

3.3   First steps

The Commission's decision to set up ECVAM was communicated to the Council and the European Parliament on 20 October 1991. Since that time, a number of steps have been taken. Firstly, two of the existing members of the staff of the Environment Institute have been assisting the director of the Institute in beginning the work of ECVAM. Secondly, a new building consisting of offices and laboratories has been planned, with building scheduled to commence early in 1993. The new facilities should be ready for occupancy by the middle of 1994.

Meanwhile, the ECVAM Scientific Advisory Committee has been formed. It consists of one representative of each of the 12 Member States, and six members selected by the Commission from individuals nominated by five organizations representative of industry, academia, and animal welfare, namely COLIPA (Comité des Associations Européenes de l'Industrie de la Parfumerie, des Produits Cosmétiques et de Toilette), ECETOC (European Chemical Industry Ecology and Toxicology Centre), EFPIA (European Federation of Pharmaceutical Industry Associations), ERGATT (European Research Group for Alternatives in Toxicity Testing), and EUROGROUP for Animal Welfare. Furthermore, Michael Balls, Chairman of the Trustees of FRAME and Professor of Medical Cell Biology at the University of Nottingham Medical School, was appointed head of ECVAM early in 1993 and took up his duties at Ispra in April. This will be followed by the appointment of other personnel with experience in alternative test methods and their validation and in the provision of information services.

3.4   Current activities

Since the SIAT Symposium, two meetings of the ECVAM Scientific Advisory Committee have taken place, one result being that the main goal of ECVAM has been redefined, as follows: *ECVAM will promote the scientific and regulatory acceptance of alternative methods which are of importance to the biosciences and which reduce, refine or replace the use of laboratory animals.* This emphasizes that ECVAM will not focus its attention merely on regulatory toxicity tests.

An ambitious program of activities is already under way, which can be summarized under the following headings: information services; workshops, task forces and symposia; external and internal projects; and training programs.

3.4.1   Information services

ECVAM is already benefiting from its collaboration with the Environmental Informatics Unit (another unit of the Environment Institute at Ispra) and with two databanks, namely the Galileo Data Bank, located at Pisa, Italy (which has an emphasis on data produced by in vitro toxicity tests), and the INVITTOX databank, located at Nottingham, U.K. (which has an emphasis on in vitro test methods). We are also planning to collaborate with the journal, *ATLA (Alternatives to Laboratory Animals)*, so that news of ECVAM's activities can be widely distributed within the scientific, industrial and animal welfare communities.

3.4.2   ECVAM workshops, task forces and symposia

One of ECVAM's first priorities must be to become well-informed about the current state-of-the-art of non-animal test development in relation to particular types of chemicals, types of products and potential toxic hazards. We are therefore planning a series of ECVAM *workshops*, in order to be able to review the current status of various types of tests and their potential uses and to identify the best ways forward.

During 1993 and early 1994, we hope to run workshops on hepatocyte culture and its uses, phototoxicology in vitro, neurotoxicity testing in vitro, in vitro screens for reproductive toxicity, and non-animal testing for corrosive chemicals. Our plans for 1994 include workshops on the integrated use of QSAR and in vitro studies, in vitro tests for dermal penetration, the use of genetically-engineered cell lines in pharmacotoxicology, the use of immortalized cells in pharmacotoxicology, and eye irritancy testing in vitro. We are also investigating the way forward with respect to vaccine potency testing, the quality control of biologicals and the testing of biomaterials.

Our strategy also involves the setting up of ECVAM *task forces* to focus on the achievement of narrowly-defined, specific goals. We see task forces as ways of implementing the recommendations of workshops in the planning of validation studies and of seeking acceptance of the outcome of successful validation studies.

ECVAM *symposia* will deal with wider issues, and at present we have only one symposium under consideration – a revisitation of the principles of validation – to mark the opening of the new ECVAM building, in September 1994.

3.4.3   ECVAM projects

It has been decided that ECVAM will have its own research and testing laboratories, which will be used for the development of new test methods, for participation in pre-validation studies and in formal validation programs, and for training courses. This decision was welcomed by the ECVAM Scientific Advisory Committee at its first meeting.

We hope to have five laboratory-based research teams by 1998, in addition to our statistical and information services. However, it is clear that ECVAM would never be able to provide expertise in all the different types of tests and areas of pharmacotoxicology for which the validation of alternative tests and test batteries will be necessary in the years to come. Collaboration with academic and industrial alternatives research laboratories in the Member States, and elsewhere, will therefore be essential.

Such collaboration is already under way. In 1993, in addition to our external contracts for information services, ECVAM will be funding pre-validation studies on in vitro phototoxicology and in vitro neurotoxicology, on the relationship between in vitro cytotoxicity and acute lethal potency, and on the further development of the ERGATT/CFN Integrated *In Vitro* Toxicity Testing Scheme (ECITTS). In addition, ECVAM will be involved in three international interlaboratory validation studies, on alternatives to the Draize eye irritancy test, on measuring inhibition of gap junction intercellular communication in vitro as a means of identifying tumor promoters, and on in vitro tests for photoirritants.

3.4.4   Training programs

Training will be a very important part of ECVAM's activities, in two main ways.

We will want to contribute to general training programs which emphasize the Three Rs approach to the proper regulation and supervision of laboratory animal procedures, as will be required in the Member States in compliance with Directive 86/609/EEC.

However, our main commitment will be to training in the principles and practice of validation, taking into account the many factors which must be considered when the reliability and relevance of a new method for a particular purpose or purposes are being assessed and challenged, e. g. in a blind trial.

Courses will also be run in collaboration with other laboratories and organizations, to contribute to the general training of in vitro pharmacotoxicologists and others or to develop competence in the application of specific test protocols.

Reference

EEC (1986) Council Directive of 24 November 1986 on the approximation of laws, regulations and administrative provisions of the Member States regarding the protection of animals used for experimental and other scientific purposes. *Official Journal of the European Communities* **29**, (L358), 1–29.

4 A Timetable for Replacing, Reducing and Refining Animal Use with the Help of in Vitro Tests: The Limulus Amebocyte Lysate Test (LAL) as an Example

Oliver Flint

Summary

Concern about progress in validating in vitro tests that might refine, reduce or replace animal use has, in recent years, generated vigorous debate about the process of test validation and acceptance. The debate has proceeded largely in the abstract without reference to actual cases. One in vitro test, the Limulus amebocyte lysate test (LAL), addresses the problem of identifying agents that cause endotoxic shock, a complex pattern of systemic toxicity. The LAL test has achieved the status of largely replacing the rabbit pyrogenicity test, formerly used in the detection of endotoxins. There are useful lessons to be learnt about the process of in vitro test development from the LAL test. The test is an extremely sensitive measure of coagulation (gelling) of Limulus blood, in the presence of endotoxin. Coagulation of Limulus (horseshoe crab) and mammalian blood is analogous in several respects. Disseminated intra-vascular coagulation (DIC) is one of the possible symptoms of endotoxic shock in Limulus and in mammals, depending on the amount of endotoxin present. Thus, the LAL test can be understood in terms of the mechanism of in vivo toxicity. However, the LAL test isolates only one of the in vivo mechanisms of toxicity. Hypotension and pyrogenicity, among other effects, are ignored.

In vitro tests, by definition, isolate specific mechanisms and behaviors of cell systems in the whole animal. This is a limitation as well as an advantage that defines how successful the test will be in its application. If the in vivo toxicity to be addressed by the in vitro test is well defined (for example DIC as a key feature of endotoxic shock) then the in vitro test may well come to reduce our reliance on animal testing methods. If the in vivo toxicity is ill defined, as is acute toxicity versus simple cytotoxicity tests, then it is unlikely that the in vitro test will ever reduce reliance on animals.

The main features of the LAL test were first described in 1964. Almost 20 years passed between first conception of this test and its final recognition by the FDA as a replacement for the rabbit pyrogenicity test. This intervening time has involved many validation studies and the development of standard reference samples of endotoxin. Most important has been the ongoing collaboration between regulatory authorities and industrial laboratories interested in applying the in vitro test. We must promote better collaboration between industrial, academic and regulatory scientists to achieve the goal of reducing animal use through the application of in vitro tests. We must also use practical examples, like the LAL test, as guides.

Alternatives to Animal Testing. New Ways in the Biomedical Sciences, Trends and Progress.
Reinhardt, C. A. (ed.). 1994. © VCH, Weinheim.

Abbreviations. DIC = disseminated intravascular coagulation; IL-1 = interleukin-1; LAL = Limulus amebocyte lysate, TNF = tumor necrosis factor.

4.1   Introduction

Many new techniques of in vitro testing for toxic hazard have been described in recent years and some have made the transition from the developer's laboratory to application in the pharmaceutical or consumer products industry (Flint, 1990a; Flint and Boyle, 1990). The process of transition, also known as technology transfer, requires that the test has been validated for its proposed use (Balls *et al.*, 1990; Flint 1990b; Flint, 1991). Validation involves demonstrating an acceptable degree of correspondance between the interpretation of the in vitro test and in vivo test results that best characterize potential human toxicity. The type of test determines to what extent validation is possible. The heuristic approach to test development has had considerable influence on the types of tests now widely available. This is best illustrated in a recent article by Flavia Zucco (1992). She develops the argument that, because mechanisms of toxicity will never be completely understood, the empirical approach is both necessary and desirable. In its most extreme form this has been described by Nardone, and also quoted by Zucco, as the "carnation test" (Nardone, 1980):

> I would like to conclude by reminding the reader that in vitro technology serves many purposes. Hence, tests which satisfy one need may not satisfy another. It is not uncommon to hear heated exchanges regarding prediction and extrapolation. Some argue that the in vitro test method must be capable of generating the toxic endpoint exactly the way it occurs in vivo. Others, recalling that the primary role of screening studies is prediction with a relatively high level of confidence, care not how the prediction can be made, as long as it is reliable. For example, let us assume that a validation study shows that many diverse neurotoxic substances added to a vase kill carnations in 90 % of the tests. The death of carnations would then be considered an acceptable endpoint for screening neurotoxic substances. While this is disquieting from an intellectual and scientific point of view, it has validity if the test has predictability and other advantages such as speed and low cost.

> It is our obligation to recognize the diverse needs of society and existing time and fiscal constraints. Society needs scientific understanding, but primarily for mechanisms, it also needs to have the large number of chemicals screened. Tissue culture can assist in both if we remain reasonable in our expectations and clear regarding the purposes of our studies.

Nardone takes the high ground between two opposing camps. In one camp are the extreme empiricists, requiring no explanation for function, and in the other the Cartesians, requiring an ordered understanding of mechanisms. Like Swift's Gulliver, Nardone calls for clarity and reason in the debate between the "Little Enders" and the "Big Enders." Unthinking acceptance of an apparently fortuitous relationship between the result of an in vitro test and some (often carefully selected) in vivo test endpoint is as absurd as the demand for a complete understanding of toxic mechanism before successful in vitro tests can be designed. The reality is that the empirical and the strictly rational approach most often go hand in hand. No clinical test could be successfully applied without an explanation of what the test involves and why the test works. Explanation, however, does not always imply a complete understanding and there may be significant empirical components to the test. The working mixture of individual components that makes an assay successful consists of various proportions of experience, trial and error, and understanding. The carnation test is 100 % trial and error. There is no guarantee that the test will continue to work effectively with future test agents. This is not adequate when human risk needs to be determined. The guarantee that future application of the test will correctly identify potentially toxic agents is provided by our understanding of the test, its mechanisms, and how they relate to affected mechanisms in vivo. Confidence in the interpretation of test results will be determined by the extent to which we understand how the test works.

Consideration of the nature of in vitro tests in the abstract helps provide some of the ground rules for their selection and application, but a concrete example provides the supporting evidence. Few in vitro assays have approached the complete replacement of an animal toxicity test. One of these assays, the Limulus amebocyte lysate (LAL) test, bears examination because it illustrates well the development and acceptance of an in vitro test. The objective of this paper is to discover some of the lessons that may be learnt from this process of development and acceptance. This is not intended to be a definitive review of the LAL test. For those seeking more complete information excellent reviews can be found in (Levin, 1985; Pearson *et al.*, 1982c; Prior, 1990).

4.2   Endotoxin

Endotoxin is a mixture of the lipopolysaccharide from the wall of Gram-negative bacteria, protein and other trace components (Elin and Wolff, 1982; Prior, 1990). Lipopolysaccharide is a complex mixture of molecules with molecular weights varying from 400 to 4000 kD (Raetz, 1990). The most conserved part of these molecules is a 2-kD fragment known as lipid A, which on its own can induce many of the features of endotoxic shock (Morrison and Ryan, 1987; Rietschel *et al.*, 1982). Bacterial contamination of medical equipment used for intravenous perfusion, water used in the preparation of intravenous injectable pharmaceuticals, or items such as the syringe used for the injection can lead to endotoxic shock. Effects vary, from mild (fever) to life threatening (blood clotting, extreme hypotension, toxic shock), depending on the amount of endotoxin present. Humans are particularly sensitive to very small amounts of endotoxin in the nanogram/ml range (Wardle, 1975). Living bacteria need not be present, and normal steam sterilization procedures are not sufficient to remove trace amounts of endotoxin contamination. Equipment and injectable solutions must be tested for the presence of endotoxin. The test originally involved using rabbits, but recently rabbit pyrogenicity (fever inducing) tests have almost completely been replaced by the more sensitive in vitro LAL test.

The major pathophysiological effects of endotoxin are mediated by cytokines and other factors released by cells of the macrophage/phagocyte system (see Figure 4-1). Endotoxin activates mononuclear phagocytes to release interleukin-1 (IL-1), which in turn acts on the hypothalamus to cause fever (Cooper *et al.*, 1967; Lipton and Kennedy, 1979; Morrison and Ryan, 1987). Monocytes carry specific membrane receptors for lipopolysaccharide (Roeder *et al.*, 1989; Wright, 1991). IL-1 can induce many other physiological responses, including the

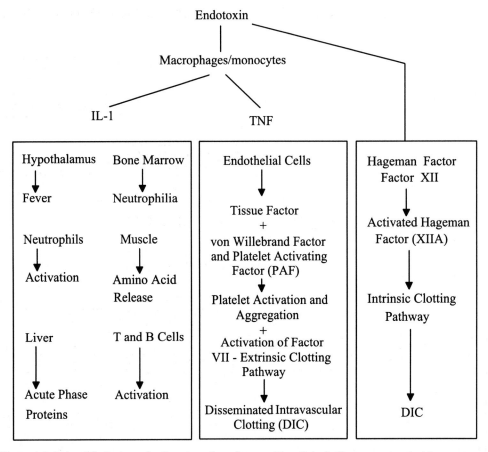

Figure 4-1. A simplified scheme for the generation of some of the clinical effects associated with exposure to endotoxin. Endotoxin activates macrophages which release IL-1 and TNF. IL-1 acts on cells in the organ systems indicated in the box to cause the clinically observed effects. Similarly TNF acts on endothelial cells lining the blood vessels to initiate the coagulation process. There is considerable overlap between the effects of TNF and IL-1 (Le and Vilcek, 1987) which is not indicated in this scheme and several other mediators are significantly involved. Intravascular clotting can be initiated by the extrinsic or the intrinsic pathways. Clotting of Limulus blood when exposed to endotoxin most closely resembles activation of the intrinsic clotting pathway in mammals.

release of acute phase proteins from the liver and neutrophilia. Activated macrophages also produce tumor necrosis factor (TNF) which enhances fibrin deposition, promotes disseminated intravascular coagulation (DIC), and reduces the anticoagulant activity of neutrophils (Matthews, 1981; Prior, 1990). Endotoxin also stimulates procoagulant activity (Morrison and Ryan, 1987) either by direct activation of Hageman factor, or by the action of monocyte released TNF on the endothelial cells of the blood vessel (secretion of tissue factor, platelet activating factor, and von Willebrand factor). Procoagulant activity may lead to DIC. The complex symptomatology of endotoxic shock is a direct result of the number of biological mediators induced and their many different effects (Cotran *et al.*, 1989; Prior, 1990). It is surprising that among all the many possible endpoints that could be used to detect the presence and activity of endotoxin, only two have formed the basis of a successful test. These are pyrogenicity in rabbits and coagulation in the LAL test.

4.3   In vivo test for pyrogenicity

Pyrogenicity following injection of various agents, including distilled water, was first described by Billroth (1865) and Burdon-Sanderson (1876). Soon after it was recognized that this was due not to contamination with living bacteria, but to a heat-stable, non-proteinaceous substance generated by bacterial cultures (Centanni, 1894). This heat-stable substance was later shown to produce fever in rabbits (Jona, 1916; Seibert, 1923, 1925; Seibert and Bourn, 1925; Seibert and Mendel, 1923). Using Gram-negative bacteria as pyrogens Hort and Penfold (1912) devised the first standard method for testing for pyrogens in rabbits. These were the foundations of the rabbit pyrogenicity test. The standardized rabbit pyrogenicity test was established in the 1940s (Co Tui and Schrift, 1942; McCloskey *et al.*, 1943) and guidelines were issued by the U. S. Pharmacopoeia and the FDA. A more complete review of the test and further references can be found in Weiss (1978), Weary and Wallin (1973) and Outschoorn (1982).

The objective of the test is to measure small changes (tenths of a degree centigrade) in rectal temperature over three or more hours following intravenous injection of a solution containing potential pyrogen or a prepared standard. Increase in body temperature above an accepted threshold ($>0.6\,°C$) is normally taken to indicate the presence of unacceptable amounts of pyrogen in the injected sample. Mature, healthy rabbits are selected and acclimatized to laboratory conditions. The numbers of animals involved are small (three to five per test). Test animal handling, conditions of restraint and prior disease status are among many factors that may influence the test result. Another important factor is reuse. Animals may be reused even if a prior response has been observed, but both tolerance or increased sensitivity may interfere with future tests. Variability in response is also related to laboratory, strain, time of day, or season (Bellentani, 1982; Kühnhold, 1977; Simon *et al.*, 1976, 1977; Van Dijk and Van de Voorde, 1977).

Variability can be controlled and is not the most important limitation of the in vivo test. The test requires a dedicated facility and trained personnel to be maintained at all times. The expense is a major limitation. The test is also inappropriate for certain classes of drugs, including short-lived radiopharmaceuticals, hypnotics, and sedatives (Cooper, 1979; Cooper and Pearson, 1977), antibiotics, which may themselves induce an allergic response (De Weck, 1983; Kraft, 1983), and plasma proteins and antigens (Ronneberger, 1977). It would also be logical to assume that the test is inappropriate for testing samples of cytokines such as IL-1 and growth factors intended for therapeutic use, which may directly induce changes in body temperature.

4.4   In vitro test for endotoxins: The LAL test

One of the most fascinating aspects of the historical development of the LAL test is that it was not discovered as a result of a directed effort to develop an alternative to the rabbit pyrogenicity test (Levin, 1985). The earliest studies showing that coagulation of the blood of *Limulus polyphemus* (Limulus), or horseshoe crab, was a comparable physiological phenomenon to the coagulation of mammalian blood were almost contemporaneous (Howell, 1885) with the earliest studies on pyrogenicity in the rabbit (Billroth, 1865). Limulus blood was observed to coagulate when brought into contact with cleaned glass. Seventy years later Bang (1956) reported a bacterial disease of Limulus that caused intravascular coagulation of the blood, similar to that seen when blood was isolated from the animal and brought into contact with glass. Within a few years an interest in the basic process of coagulation led Levin (Levin and Bang, 1964) to the observation that Limulus blood would not coagulate on pyrogen free glassware, the confirmation that endotoxin was responsible for coagulation (Levin and Bang, 1968), and the description of a standard test method (Cooper et al., 1971). It was the need for a test for pyrogenic contamination of short-lived radionuclides used as radiocontrast agents that initially led to the more widespread acceptance of the LAL test as an alternative to the rabbit pyrogenicity test (Cooper and Harbert, 1976). Between 1970 and 1976, however, there was sufficient medical application of the LAL test in the detection of endotoxin that the FDA (Bureau of Biologics), which had been investigating the test for its own needs, had already begun to regulate its use (Federal Register, 1973; Hochstein, 1990).

The FDA did not release its final guideline on the LAL test, accepting its use as an alternative to the rabbit pyrogenicity test, until almost 20 years after the discovery that endotoxin caused coagulation (U. S. D. H. H. S., 1987; see Figure 4-3). Three different types of studies were done during this time to standardize and validate the LAL test. First, the sensitivity of the LAL test to the presence of lipopolysaccharide in a wide variety of samples was established (Table 4-1). Secondly, there was a major international effort comparing the LAL and the rabbit pyrogenicity test (Table 4-2). Thirdly, a standard endotoxin sample was developed as a positive control for the LAL test (Csako et al., 1983; Poole and Mussett, 1989; Weidner et al., 1987).

All of the factors necessary for coagulation in Limulus blood are contained within the amebocytes, its major class of blood cell (Levin and Bang, 1964, 1968). The LAL test therefore requires a lysate prepared from amebocytes. There are a number of licensed manufacturers of the lysate in the United States (Hochstein, 1990). The manufacturer collects samples of blood from horseshoe crabs that are then returned unharmed to the sea (Prior, 1990). Lysate is divided up into aliquots and lyophilized prior to storage. Stored samples can be used up to one year after preparation, even when kept at room temperature (Prior, 1990). Components of the lysate required for coagulation are a proclotting enzyme, a clottable protein, and calcium ions. An essential step in endotoxin-induced coagulation is activation of the proclotting enzyme (Figure 4-2). Coagulation can be observed one hour after mixing the lysate with an endotoxin containing sample. Coagulation is an all or none endpoint. The time can be considerably reduced to 10 minutes or less, and the endpoint can be transformed into a quantitative assay for endotoxin if a chromogenic substrate is included as an indicator of proclotting enzyme activation. Very small quantities of sample can be tested ranging from 100 to 200 μl of sample and lysate in the standard test (Prior, 1990) to as little as 1 μl of each in a modification of the test using glass capillaries (Gardi and Arpagaus, 1980). The sensitivity is extremely high, permitting detection of as little as 1 pg of endotoxin (Cooper, 1990; Friberger, 1985).

There are clear analogies between the clotting of Limulus blood and the intrinsic pathway of mammalian blood coagulation, though the former is much simpler than the latter. There is a cascade of biochemical events leading to amplification of the response. Activation of clotting factors (C and B in Limulus, Factor XII in mammals) is required to initiate the cas-

Table 4-1. Typical applications of the Limulus amebocyte lysate test in the detection of endotoxin.

Application	Reference
Parenteral injectable products (distilled water, dextrose, saline, mannitol, electrolyte solutions, etc.)	Mascoli and Weary, 1979 Tsuji *et al.*, 1980 Cooper, 1990
Blood products (whole blood, plasma, serum albumin, immunoglobulin, antihemophilic factor, etc.)	McCleod and Katz, 1981 Hochstein and Seligman, 1979 Homma *et al.*, 1982 Cundell *et al.*, 1982
Medical devices (transfusion and infusion assemblies, dyalysis equipment, packaging components for parenteral products, etc.)	Pearson *et al.*, 1982a Ross and Bruch, 1982 Henne *et al.*, 1984 Pearson *et al.*, 1987 Helme, 1982
Radiopharmaceutical preparations (hemodynamic tracers, radiocontrasting agents, etc.)	Cooper and Harbert, 1975 Bruneau *et al.*, 1986 Cohen *et al.*, 1986
Antibiotics (aminoglycosides, cephalosporins, penicillins, etc.)	Harrison *et al.*, 1979 McCullough, 1982 Case *et al.*, 1983 Al-Khalifa *et al.*, 1989
Detection of bacterial infection in body fluids other than blood (cerebrospinal fluid, urine, synovial fluid, etc.)	Munford *et al.*, 1984 Nachum, 1990 Elin, 1990

Table 4-2. References illustrating the international validation of the LAL test in comparison with the rabbit pyrogenicity test.

Country	Reference
United States	Eibert, 1972 Wachtel and Tsuji, 1977 Tsuji *et al.*, 1980 Weary *et al.*, 1980, 1982 Pearson *et al.*, 1982b Kleszynski *et al.*, 1982
Germany (DDR)	Ronneberger and Stärk, 1974 Ronneberger, 1977 Godau, 1980 Richter *et al.*, 1980 Müller-Calgan, 1982
France	Cohen *et al.*, 1986 Bruneau *et al.*, 1986
Netherlands	Van Noordwijk, 1979 Bleeker *et al.*, 1985
Japan	Kanoh and Kawasaki, 1980 Kanoh, 1982
Hungary	Nyerges and Jaszovszky, 1981

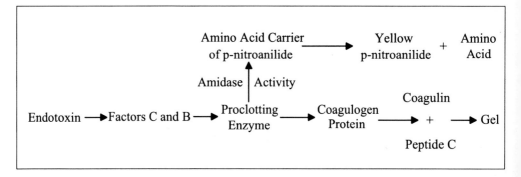

Figure 4-2. Key mechanisms involved in the Limulus amebocyte lysate (LAL) gel and chromogenic tests (adapted from Prior, 1990). Factors essential for clotting in the lysate are Factors C and B, proclotting enzyme and the clottable protein, coagulogen. Endotoxin interacts with Factors C and B to activate the proclotting enzyme. In the gel test, the proclotting enzyme cleaves coagulogen into coagulin and C-peptide chains. Peptide chains cross-link by hydrophobic or hydrophilic interactions and a gel matrix or clot is formed. Gel formation takes approximately 1 hr. In the chromogenic test, advantage is taken of the amidase activity of the proclotting enzyme which cleaves yellow colored p-nitroanilide from an amino acid carrier. Optimum color formation is observed 10 min after starting the reaction.

cade. Some of the same enzymatic inhibitors block mammalian and horseshoe crab coagulation, and synthetic substrates designed for the assay of human coagulation factors are also substrates for the components of the Limulus coagulation system (reviewed by Fujita and Nakahara, 1982 and Levin, 1985). Coagulation of blood is not the only in vivo response to endotoxin but is to be expected following exposure to sufficiently high quantities of endotoxin (Prior, 1990). The LAL test, like the rabbit pyrogenicity test, does not predict every possible outcome of exposure to endotoxin. Instead it measures a universal property of endotoxin which may or may not be observed in vivo depending on the conditions of exposure and the amount of endotoxin involved.

4.5   Major steps in the evolution of an in vitro test

A review of some of the major milestones in the development of the LAL test (Figure 4-3) reveals that it took more than a century from the first description of pyrogenicity to the regulatory acceptance of an in vitro test for endotoxin. The tests arose independently from one another and it was not before recognition of the involvement of endotoxin in both pyrogenicity and Limulus blood coagulation that the idea for a test involving Limulus amebocyte lysate arose. There is thus a second, much shorter time line, starting with the idea for the LAL test and ending in its final acceptance as an alternative to the rabbit pyrogenicity test. Interestingly, this period of 20 years is similar to the time between first observation of endotoxin-induced pyrogenicity in rabbits and the acceptance of a standardized rabbit pyrogen test.

Figure 4-3 confirms one obvious conclusion. The bulk of experimental work in animals defining the pathophysiological reponse to endotoxin was required before the LAL test could be developed. In general, this suggests that an understanding of the underlying nature of toxicity is an essential component of in vitro test development.

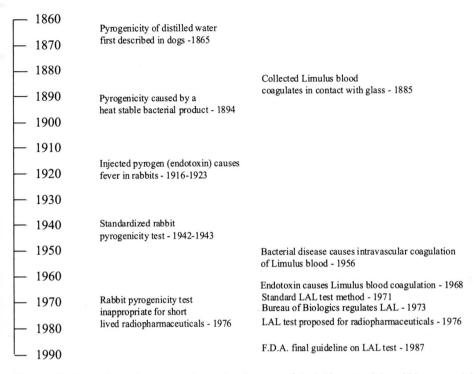

1860

Pyrogenicity of distilled water
first described in dogs -1865

1870

1880

Collected Limulus blood
coagulates in contact with glass - 1885

1890

Pyrogenicity caused by a
heat stable bacterial product - 1894

1900

1910

Injected pyrogen (endotoxin) causes
fever in rabbits - 1916-1923

1920

1930

1940

Standardized rabbit
pyrogenicity test - 1942-1943

1950

Bacterial disease causes intravascular coagulation
of Limulus blood - 1956

1960

Endotoxin causes Limulus blood coagulation - 1968
Standard LAL test method - 1971
Bureau of Biologics regulates LAL - 1973

1970

Rabbit pyrogenicity test
inappropriate for short
lived radiopharmaceuticals - 1976

LAL test proposed for radiopharmaceuticals - 1976

1980

F.D.A. final guideline on LAL test - 1987

1990

Figure 4-3. Comparison of milestones in the development of the LAL test and the rabbit pyrogenicity test.

4.6 Discussion

One of the most significant lessons to be learned from the rabbit pyrogenicity test and the LAL test for endotoxin is that each only measures one isolated aspect of endotoxin toxicity. A test designed from a complete understanding of the mechanism of endotoxin induced toxicity was not required to detect the presence of endotoxin. Nevertheless, these tests are by no means carnation tests, as described by Nardone (1980). The endpoints measured are directly related to the mechanism of action of endotoxin. The relevance of these effects (pyrogenicity in the rabbit, coagulation of Limulus blood) to endotoxic shock was accepted before the validity of the tests was recognized. The LAL test has all the essential features of an in vitro test: speed, ease of use, size of sample, reproducibility, and standardization. Mechanistic relevance is an additional feature which has not often been mentioned and which some authors (e. g. Balls *et al.*, 1990; Zucco, 1992) have explicitly excluded as an absolute requirement. Without demonstration of mechanistic relevance the LAL test would never have been adopted as an acceptable alternative to the rabbit pyrogenicity test. The importance of this point cannot be underestimated. Human safety is the objective of eliminating endotoxin contamination. Human safety requires a guarantee that the test identifies a toxic agent by mechanisms that are understood to be related to toxicity in vivo. A carnation test does not provide this guarantee. A successful test, such as the LAL test, fulfills the objectives of reducing, refining and replacing animals in medical experiments, but this is not its primary objective. Human safety is the primary objective (Flint, 1992).

The conclusions reached so far in this discussion may seem to have been sufficiently self-evident not to have required discussion at all. In a recent article, Zucco (1992) dismisses this type of conclusion as equivalent to the self-evident humor of an Italian comedian, Catalano. The point of using the self-evident in humor is, sadly, its lack of self-evidence for many people. For example, Zucco asks whether massive failure of basal cellular functions causing functional disruption of an organ or tissue is not also a sufficient explanation of acute toxicity (Zucco, 1992). This hypothesis has been the basis of major in vitro toxicity effort. At least two international studies, the Multicenter Evaluation of In Vitro Cytotoxicity (MEIC) and the FRAME multicenter project on in vitro toxicology, have compared the cytotoxic behavior of a number of chemicals with their known in vivo toxicity (Bondesson et al., 1989; Ekwall et al., 1989; Knox, 1986; Mazziotti, 1990; Zanetti et al., 1992). One of these, the MEIC study, is still ongoing. Many independent studies have assumed the hypothesis (Babich and Borenfreund, 1990; Ekwall, 1981, 1983; Ekwall and Acosta, 1982; Halle and Spielmann, 1992; Peloux et al., 1992; Stammati et al., 1981; Walum and Peterson, 1984). Balls et al. (1990), in their comprehensive discussion of in vitro test validation, assume this hypothesis and the necessity of carnation tests. The extreme result of endotoxic shock is death. Massive failure of basal cellular functions is certainly involved at the end. Among the initial mechanisms involved, however, is receptor mediated excretion of cytokines leading to fever, hypotension, and DIC. These are the mechanisms that need to be isolated in the culture dish. This argument is not specific to endotoxin but, with the possible exception of toxins that poison respiration (for example, cyanide), is generally applicable. Even in the case of cyanide, there is little direct correlation between death of the animal and cell death in tissue culture. Potassium cyanide interrupts the mitochondrial electron transport chain and alone can only deplete cellular ATP in cultured cells to between 30 and 50 % control values (Maduh et al., 1991). Complete chemical anoxia can only be achieved in the presence of cyanide plus an inhibitor of glycolysis such as iodoacetate (Nicotera et al., 1989). Under argon atmosphere-induced hypoxic conditions cultured cells survive cyanide exposure better than in air (Aw and Jones, 1989). Cultured cells can thus survive chemical or atmospheric hypoxia by using glycolysis, and the resultant reduction in dependence on mitochondrial respiration renders the cell less, not more, sensitive to cyanide poisoning. In vivo, the rapid death of the animal is not explained by general suppression of cellular respiration, leading to hypoxia. The animal dies rapidly following direct central suppression of respiration (breathing). Other factors such as stimulation of a massive release of catecholamines from the adrenal chromaffin cells are also involved in acute cyanide toxicity (Kanthasamy et al., 1991a, 1991b). The attempt to identify the consequences (death of the whole animal) with the behavior of cells in the culture dish (cell death) is a profound mistake. Worse, it presents us with a comfortable and oversimplified explanation of toxicity while discouraging a pressing need to devote our efforts to the pursuit of better explanations.

Another significant lesson to be learnt is that the time required to develop an in vitro test and to obtain widespread acceptance of its use depends on many factors, some of which are not easy to control. Most important among these factors is the perceived need for the test. The rabbit pyrogenicity test was inappropriate for certain products, including short-lived radiopharmaceuticals, yet endotoxic shock was observed to be a major problem. There was thus a significant human safety factor involved in the acceptance of the LAL test. It was fortunate that studies on endotoxin-induced Limulus blood coagulation were successfully under way at the same time that this need became pressing. Thus, the LAL test had a very rapid passage from its early development to widespread use. The final recognition of this in vitro test by regulatory authorities, such as the FDA, as an accredited alternative to the rabbit pyrogenicity test has taken much longer. Three principal requirements had to be met before the test could be accepted as part of the regulatory guidelines. The test had to be standardized and an internationally recognized standard positive control developed. Validation studies were needed to compare the rabbit pyrogenicity test with the LAL test, and many different kinds of products had to be tested to define the limitations of the LAL test. There was no preliminary announcement by the regulatory authorities that these requirements had to be met. Nevertheless there was active collaboration between the regulatory authorities, clinical scientists seeking a better understanding of the test, and industries developing the test for practical application. The LAL test is thus a test case defining the requirements for acceptance by regulatory authorities that should be met by all in vitro tests.

In summary, the requirements for an in vitro test that will be accepted by the scientific community and the regulatory authorities as a useful alternative to animal testing are as follows:

– A demonstrable need for the test.
– An understanding of the mechanisms involved in the identification of toxic agents by the test that is sufficient to establish a strong relationship with the mechanisms underlying toxicity in vivo.
– Clearly defined endpoints that can be interpreted in terms of an equivalent effect in vivo. Some examples are: transport of organic ions across a monolayer of kidney proximal tubule cells, induction or inhibition of identified isotypes of cytochrome P450 in hepatocytes, inhibition of myocyte beat rate via specific receptor binding, inhibition of axonal transport in fascicles of cultured dorsal root ganglion cells.
– Avoidance of lack of precision, or clear definition of what is being measured and its relationship to toxicity in vivo. For example, the cytotoxicity endpoint using cell lines has, at different times, been proposed as an assay for acute toxicity in vivo (references quoted in preceding discussion), reproductive hazard (Pratt and Willis, 1985), acute neurotoxicity (Walum and Peterson, 1983), ocular (reviewed in Frazier *et al.*, 1987), dermal (Babich *et al.*, 1989), or kidney toxicity (Linseman *et al.*, 1990).
– Standardization of the test method.
– A standard positive control giving a defined response in the test.
– Wide validation of the test using many different classes of test agents with known in vivo toxicity, establishing test limitations.
– Collaboration between regulatory, academic and industrial scientists.
– Defininition of the variability that may be induced by factors such as test material or reagent preparation.
– Sufficient time for all the conditions listed above to have been met satisfactorily.

References

Al-Khalifa I. J., Naidu N. V., Nallari V. R. and Raut H. I. (1989) Effect of some penicillins on the sensitivity of Limulus Amebocyte Lysate test. *Journal of Pharmacy and Pharmacology* **41**, 127–128.

Aw T. Y. and Jones D. P. (1989) Cyanide toxicity in hepatocytes under aerobic and anaerobic conditions. *American Journal of Physiology* **257**, C435–441.

Babich H. and Borenfreund E. (1990) Applications of the neutral red cytotoxicity assay to in vitro toxicology. *ATLA* **18**, 129–144.

Babich H., Martin-Alguacil N. and Borenfreund E. (1989) Comparisons of the cytotoxicities of dermatotoxicants to human keratinocytes and fibroblasts in vitro. In *Alternative Methods in Toxicology, Vol. 7. In Vitro Toxicology: New Directions.* Edited by A. M. Goldberg. pp. 153–167. Mary Ann Liebert, Inc., New York.

Balls M., Blaauboer B., Brusick D., Frazier J., Lamb D., Pemberton M., Reinhardt C., Roberfroid M., Rosenkrantz H., Schmid B., Spielmann H., Stammati A.-L. and Walum E. (1990) Report and recommendations of the CAAT/ERGATT workshop on the validation of toxicity test procedures. *ATLA* **18**, 313–317.

Bang F. B. (1956) A bacterial disease of Limulus polyphemus. *Bulletin of the Johns Hopkins Hospital* **98**, 325–351.

Bellentani L. (1982) Cyclic and chronobiological considerations when employing the rabbit fever test. *Progress in Clinical and Biological Research* **93**, 329–342.

Billroth T. (1865) Beobachtung-Studien über Wundfieber und accidentelle Wundkrankheiten. *Archiv für klinische Chirurgie* **6**, 372–495.

Bleeker W. K., Kannegieter E. M., Bakker J. C. and Loos J. A. (1985) Endotoxin in blood products: correlation between the Limulus assay and the rabbit pyrogen test. *Progress in Clinical and Biological Research* **189**, 293–303.

Bondesson I., Ekwall B., Hellberg S., Romert L., Stenberg K. and Walum E. (1989). MEIC A new international multicenter project to evaluate the relevance to human toxicity of in vitro cytotoxicity tests. *Cell Biology and Toxicology* **5**, 331–348.

Bruneau J., Cohen Y., Merlin L. and Peysson S. (1986) La recherche des endotoxines dans les préparations radiopharmaceutiques II. Comparaison de la sensibilité des methodes utilisant le lapin et le lysat d'amebocytes de Limule pour la détection d'endotoxines. *International Journal of Nuclear Medicine and Biology* **12**, 471–476.

Burdon-Sanderson J. (1876) On the process of fever. *Practitioner* **16**, 257–280, 337–358, 417–431.

Case M. J., Ryther S. S. and Novitsky T. J. (1983) Detection of endotoxin in antibiotic solutions with Limulus amebocyte lysate. *Antimicrobial Agents and Chemotherapy* **23**, 649–652.

Centanni E. (1894) Ueber Infektions-Fieber. *Chemisches Zentralblatt* (4th series) **6**, 597.

Co Tui F. W. and Schrift M. H. (1942) A tentative test for pyrogen in infusion fluids. *Proceedings of the Society for Experimental Biology and Medicine* **49**, 320–323.

Cohen Y., Bahri F., Bruneau J., Dubuis M., Merlin L., Michaud T. and Peysson S. (1986) La recherche des endotoxines dans les préparations radiopharmaceutiques III. Validation du test Limulus sur les préparations radiopharmaceutiques; corrélation avec l'essai des pyrogènes sur le lapin. *International Journal of Nuclear Medicine and Biology* **12**, 477–481.

Cooper J. F. (1979) Acceptance of the Limulus test as an alternative pyrogen test for radiopharmaceutical and intrathecal drugs. *Progress in Clinical and Biological Research* **29**, 345–352.

Cooper J. F. (1990) Evaluation of sterile pharmaceuticals and medical devices: An overview. In *Clinical Applications of the Limulus Amebocyte Lysate Test.* Edited by R. B. Prior. pp. 159–166. CRC Press, Boca Raton.

Cooper J. F. and Harbert J. C. (1975) Endotoxin as a cause of aseptic meningitis after radionuclide cisternography. *Journal of Nuclear Medicine* **16**, 809–815.

Cooper J. F., Levin J. and Wagner H. W. (1971) Quantitative comparison of in vitro and in vivo methods for the detection of endotoxin. *Journal of Laboratory and Clinical Medicine* **78**, 138–148.

Cooper J. F. and Pearson S. M. (1977) Detection of endotoxin in biological products by the Limulus test. *Developments in Biological Standardization* **34**, 713.

Cooper K. E., Cranston W. I., and Honour A. J. (1967) Observations on the site and mode of action of pyrogens in the rabbit brain. *Journal of Physiology* (London) **191**, 325–337.

Cotran R. S., Kumar V. and Robbins S. L. (1989). Chapter 2. Inflammation and repair. Chapter 3. Fluid and hemodynamic derangements. *Robbins Patholic Basis of Disease*, pp. 39–120. W. B. Saunders Company, Philadelphia.

Csako G., Elin R. J., Hochstein H. D. and Tsai C.-M. (1983) Physical and biological properties of U. S. Standard Endotoxin EC after exposure to ionizing radiation. *Infection and Immunity* **41**, 190–196.

Cundell A. M., Spiegelman S. and Stryker M. H. (1982) Use of the Limulus Amebocyte Lysate endotoxin assay in plasma fractionation. *Progress in Clinical and Biological Research* **93**, 269–280.

De Weck A. L. (1983) Penicillins and cephalosporins. In *Allergic Reactions to Drugs*. Edited by A. L. De Weck and H. Bundgaard. pp. 423–482. Springer-Verlag, Berlin.

Eibert J. (1972) Pyrogen testing: Horseshoe crabs versus rabbits. *Bulletin of the Parenteral Drug Association* **26**, 253–260.

Ekwall B. (1981) Preliminary studies on the validity of in vitro measurement of drug toxicity using HeLa cells. IV. Therapeutic effects and side effects of 50 drugs related to the HeLa toxicity of the therapeutic concentrations. *Toxicology Letters* **7**, 359–366.

Ekwall B. (1983) Correlation between cytotoxicity in vitro and LD_{50} values. *Acta Pharmacologica et Toxicologica* **52**, 80–99.

Ekwall B. and Acosta D. (1982) In vitro comparative toxicity of selected drugs and chemicals in HeLa cells, Chang liver cells and rat hepatocytes. *Drug and Chemical Toxicology* **5**, 219–231.

Ekwall B., Bondesson I., Castell J. V., Gomez-Lechon M. J., Hellberg J., Jover R., Ponsoda X., Romert L., Stenberg K. and Walum E. (1989) Cytotoxicity evaluation of the first ten MEIC chemicals: Acute lethal toxicity in man predicted by cytotoxicity in five cellular assays and by oral LD50 tests in rodents. *ATLA* **17**, 83–100.

Elin R. J. (1990) Evaluation of pyrogenic arthritis. In *Clinical Applications of the Limulus Amebocyte Lysate Test*. Edited by R. B. Prior. pp. 111–114. CRC Press, Boca Raton.

Elin R. J. and Wolff S. M. (1982) Bacterial endotoxin. In *Microbial Composition: CRC Handbook of Microbiology, Vol. 4. Carbohydrates, Lipids and Minerals* (2nd ed.). Edited by I. Luskin and H. A. Lechevalier. pp. 253–281. CRC Press, Boca Raton.

Federal Register Notice, Limulus Amebocyte Lysate (Additional Standards) (38 FR 180), September 18, 1973. National Archives of the U. S., Washington.

Flint O. P. (1990a). In vitro alternatives to ocular toxicity testing: Report of a meeting organized by the Industrial In Vitro Toxicology Group. *In Vitro Toxicology* **3**, 281–291.

Flint O. P. (1990b) In vitro toxicity testing: Purpose, validation and strategy. *ATLA* **18**, 11–18.

Flint O. P. (1991) In vitro test validation. *ATLA* **19**, 140–142.

Flint O. P. (1992) In vitro toxicity testing: Redefining our objectives. *ATLA* **20**, 571–574.

Flint O. P. and Boyle F. T. (1990) Structure-teratogenicity relationships among antifungal triazoles. In *Handbook of Experimental Pharmacology, Vol. 96. Chemotherapy of Fungal Diseases*. Edited by J. F. Ryley. pp. 231–249. Springer-Verlag, Berlin.

Frazier J. M., Gad S. C., Goldberg A. M. and McCulley J. P. (Editors) (1987) *A Critical Evaluation of Alternatives to Acute Ocular Irritation Testing*. Mary Ann Liebert Inc., New York.

Friberger P. (1985) The design of a reliable endotoxin test. *Progress in Clinical and Biological Research* **189**, 139–149.

Fujita Y. and Nakahara C. (1982) Preparation and application of a new endotoxin determination kit, PYRODICK, using a chromogenic substrate. *Progress in Clinical and Biological Research* **93**, 173–182.

Gardi A. and Arpagaus G. R. (1980) Improved microtechnique for endotoxin assay by the Limulus Amebocyte Lysate test. *Analytical Biochemistry* **109**, 382–385.

Godau H. (1980) Differences in the pyrogenicity of pyrogen containing solutions after intravenous and subcutaneous application in rabbits and evidence of equally sufficient amounts of pyrogens in the Limulus Amebocyte Lysate test. *Arbeiten aus dem Paul-Ehrlich-Institut, dem Georg-Speyer-Haus und dem Ferdinand-Blum-Institut zu Frankfurt a. M.* **74**, 56–96.

Halle W. and Spielmann H. (1992) Two procedures for the prediction of acute toxicity (LD50) from cytotoxicity data. *ATLA* **20**, 40–49.

Hansen E. W. and Christensen J. D. (1990) Comparison of cultured human mononuclear cells, Limulus amebocyte lysate and rabbits in the detection of pyrogens. *Journal of Clinical Pharmacy and Therapeutics* **15**, 425–433.

Harrison S. J., Tsuji K. and Enzinger R. M. (1979) Application of LAL for detection of endotoxin in antibiotic preparations. *Progress in Clinical and Biological Research* **29**, 353–365.

Helme E. J. (1982) A method for determining pyrogen burden on packaging components. *Progress in Clinical and Biological Research* **93**, 101–104.

Henne W., Schulze H., Pelger M., Tretzel J. and Von Sengbusch G. (1984) Hollow-fiber dialyzers and their pyrogenicity testing by Limulus amebocyte lysate. *Artificial Organs* **8**, 299–305.

Hochstein H. D. (1990) Role of the FDA in regulating the Limulus Amebocyte Lysate test. In *Clinical Applications of the Limulus Amebocyte Lysate Test*. Edited by R. B. Prior. pp. 37–50. CRC Press, Boca Raton.

Hochstein H. D. and Seligman E. B. (1979) Limulus lysate testing of biologics requirements for the rabbit pyrogen test. *Progress in Clinical and Biological Research* **29**, 501–506.

Homma R., Kuratsuka K. and Akama K. (1982) Application of the LAL test and the chromogenic substrate test to the detection of endotoxin in human blood products. *Progress in Clinical and Biological Research* **93**, 301–317.

Hort E. and Penfold W. J. (1912) The reaction of salvarsan fever to other forms of injection fever. *Proceedings of the Royal Society of Medicine* (Pt III. Pathology) **5**, 131–139.

Howell W. H. (1885) Observations upon the chemical composition and coagulation of the blood of Limulus polyphemus, Callinectes hastatus, and Cucumaria sp. *Johns Hopkins University Circ.* **5**, 45.

Jona J. L. (1916) A contribution to the experimental study of fever. *Journal of Hygiene* (Cambridge) **15**, 169–194.

Kanoh S. (1982) Pyrogen test and Limulus test: On the relationship between the two tests. *Eisei Shikenjo Hokoku* **100**, 20–33.

Kanoh S. and Kawasaki H. (1980) Studies on the relationship between the pyrogen test and Limulus test. *Eisei Shikenjo Hokoku* **98**, 76–70.

Kanthasamy A. G., Borowitz J. L. and Isom G. E. (1991a) Cyanide-induced increases in plasma catecholamines: relationship to acute toxicity. *Neurotoxicology* **12**, 777–784.

Kanthasamy A. G., Maduh E. U., Peoples R. W., Borowitz J. L. and Isom G. E. (1991b) Calcium mediation of cyanide-induced catecholamine release: Implications for neurotoxicity. *Toxicology and Applied Pharmacology* **110**, 275–82.

Kleszynski R. R., Hoffman D., Odeneal A. and Aldred J. P. (1982) Apparent influence of adrenocorticotrophic hormone (ACTH) in the USP rabbit pyrogen test and evaluation of LAL as an alternative procedure. *Progress in Clinical Biology Research* **93**, 357–363.

Knox P., Uphill P. F., Fry J. R., Benford J. and Balls M. (1986) The FRAME multicenter project on in vitro cytotoxicology. *Food and Chemical Toxicology* **24**, 457–463.

Kraft D. (1983) Other antibiotics. In *Allergic Reactions to Drugs*. Edited by A. L. De Weck and H. Bundgaard. pp. 483–520. Springer-Verlag, Berlin.

Kühnhold B. (1977) Comparability of pyrogen tests. *Developments in Biological Standardization* **34**, 65–71.

Le J. and Vilcek J. (1987) Tumor necrosis factor and interleukin-1: Cytokines with multiple overlapping biological activities. *Laboratory Investigation* **56**, 234–248.

Levin J. (1985) The history of the development of the Limulus Amebocyte Lysate test. In *Bacterial Endotoxins: Structure, Biomedical Significance, and Detection with the Limulus Amebocyte Lysate Test*. Edited by J. W. Cate, H. R. Buller, A. Sturk and J. Levin. pp. 3–28. Alan R. Liss, New York.

Levin J. and Bang F. B. (1964) The role of endotoxin in the extracellular coagulation of Limulus blood. *Bulletin of the Johns Hopkins Hospital* **115**, 265–274.

Levin J. and Bang F. B. (1968) Clottable protein in Limulus: Its localization and kinetics of its coagulation by endotoxin. *Thrombosis et Diathesis Haemorrhagica* **19**, 186–197.

Linseman D. A., Raczniak T. J., Aaron C. S. and Bacon, J. A. (1990) Comparative cytotoxicity rankings of four aminoglycoside antibiotics in the Chang, SIRC and LLC-PK1 cell lines. *ATLA* **18**, 283–290.

Lipton J. M. and Kennedy J. I. (1979) Central thermosensitivity during fever produced by intr-PO/AH and intravenous injection of pyrogen. *Brain Research Bulletin* **4**, 23–24.

Maduh E. U., Borowitz J. L. and Isom G. E. (1991) Cyanide-induced alteration of the adenylate energy pool in a rat neurosecretory cell line. *Journal of Applied Toxicology* **11**, 97–101.

Mascoli C. C. and Weary M. E. (1979) Applications and advantages of the Limulus Amebocyte Lysate (LAL) pyrogen test for parenteral injectable products. *Progress in Clinical and Biological Research* **29**, 387–402.

Matthews N. (1981) Tumour necrosis factor from the rabbit. V. Synthesis in vitro by mononuclear phagocytes from various tissues of normal and BCG-injected rabbits. *British Journal of Cancer* **44**, 418–424.

Mazziotti I., Stammati A.-L. and Zucco F. (1990) In vitro cytotoxicity of 26 coded chemicals to HEp-2 cells: A validation study. *ATLA* **17**, 401–406.

McCleod C. and Katz W. (1981) A rapid method for the detection of Gram-negative bacterial endotoxins in whole blood. *Journal of Biological Standardization* **9**, 299–306.

McCloskey W. T., Price C. W., Van Winkle W., Welch H. and Calver H. O. (1943) Results of first USP collaborative study of pyrogens. *Journal of the American Pharmaceutical Association* (Scientific edition) **22**, 69–73.

McCullough K. Z. (1982) The use of LAL as an alternative to the CFR rabbit pyrogen test for disodium ticarcillin. *Progress in Clinical and Biological Research* **93**, 91–100.

Morrison D. C. and Ryan J. L. (1987) Endotoxin and disease mechanisms. *Annual Review of Medicine* **38**, 417–432.

Müller-Calgan H. (1982) Experience with comparative examinations for pyrogens by rabbit pyrogen test versus the LAL test. *Progress in Clinical and Biological Research* **93**, 343–356.

Munford R. S., Hall C. L. and Grimm L. (1984) Detection of free endotoxin in cerebrospinal fluid by the Limulus lysate test. *Infection and Immunity* **45**, 531–533.

Nachum R. (1990) Detection of Gram-negative bacteriuria. In *Clinical Applications of the Limulus Amebocyte Lysate Test*. Edited by R. B. Prior. pp. 81–96. CRC Press, Boca Raton.

Nardone R. M. (1980) The interface of toxicology and tissue culture and reflections on the carnation test. *Toxicology* **17**, 105–107.

Nicotera P., Thor H. and Orrenius S. (1989) Cytosolic-free Ca^{++} and cell killing in hepatoma 1c1c7 cells exposed to chemical anoxia. *FASEB Journal* **3**, 59–64.

Nyerges G. and Jaszovszky I. (1981) Reliability of the rabbit pyrogen test and the Limulus test in predicting the pyrogenicity of vaccines in man. *Acta microbiologica Academiae scientiarum Hungicae* **28**, 235–243.

Outschoorn A. S. (1982) The USP bacterial endotoxins test. *Progress in Clinical and Biological Research* **93**, 33–38.

Pearson F. C., Caruana R., Burkart J., Katz D. V., Chenoweth D., Dubczak J., Bohon J. and Weary M. (1987) The use of the Limulus Amebocyte Lysate assay to monitor hemodialyzer-associated soluble cellulosic material (LAL-reactive material). *Progress in Clinical and Biological Research* **231**, 211–222.

Pearson F. C., Weary M. E. and Bohon J. (1982a) Detection of Limulus amebocyte lysate reactive material in capillary flow hemodialyzers. *Progress in Clinical and Biological Research* **93**, 247–260.

Pearson F. C., Weary M. E., Bohon J. and Dabbah R. (1982b) Relative potency of "environmental" endotoxin as measured by the Limulus Amebocyte Lysate test and the USP rabbit pyrogen test. *Progress in Clinical and Biological Research* **93**, 65–77.

Pearson F. C., Weary M. E. and Dabbah R. (1982c) A corporate approach to in-process and end-product testing with the LAL assay for endotoxin. In *Endotoxins and Their Detection with the Limulus Amebocyte Lysate Test*. Edited by S. W. Watson, J. Levin and T. J. Novitsky. pp. 231–246. Alan R. Liss, New York.

Peloux A.-F., Fédérici C., Bichet N., Gouy D. and Cano J.-P. (1992) Hepatocytes in primary culture: An alternative to LD50 testing? Validation of a predictive model by multivariate analysis. *ATLA* **20**, 8–26.

Poole S. and Mussett M. V. (1989) The international standard for endotoxin: Evaluation in an international collaborative study. *Journal of Biological Standardization* **17**, 161–171.

Pratt R. M. and Willis W. D. (1985) Prescreening for environmental teratogens using cultured mesenchymal cells from the human embryonic palate. *Teratogenesis, Carcinogenesis, and Mutagenesis* **2**, 313–318.

Prior R. B. (1990) The Limulus Amebocyte Lysate test. In *Clinical Applications of the Limulus Amebocyte Lysate Test*. Edited by R. B. Prior. pp. 27–36. CRC Press, Boca Raton.

Raetz C. R. H. (1990) Biochemistry of endotoxins. *Annual Review of Biochemistry* **59**, 129–170.

Richter K., Grahlow W.-D. and Wigert R. (1980) Ein Beitrag zum Vergleich des Limulustests mit dem Pyrogentest am Kanninchen. *Acta biologica et medica Germanica* **39**, 277–280.

Rietschel E. T., Galanos C., Luderitz O. and Westphal O. (1982) The chemistry and biology of lipopolysaccharides and their lipid A component. In *Immunopharmacology and the Regulation of Leukocyte Function*. Edited by D. R. Webb. pp. 183–193. Marcel Dekker, New York.

Roeder D. J., Lei M. G. and Morrison D. C. (1989) Endotoxic-lipopolysaccharide-specific binding proteins on lymphoid cells of various animal species: association with endotoxin susceptibility. *Infection and Immunity* **57**, 1054–1058.

Ronneberger H. J. (1977) Comparison of the pyrogen tests in rabbits and with Limulus lysate. *Developments in Biological Standardization* **34**, 27–36.

Ronneberger H. J. and Stärk J. (1974) Der Limulustest im Vergleich mit dem Pyrogentest am Kaninchen. *Arzneimittel-Forschung* **24**, 933–934.

Ross V. C. and Bruch C. W. (1982) Endotoxin testing of medical devices with LAL: FDA requirements. *Progress in Clinical and Biological Research* **93**, 39–48.

Seibert F. B. (1923) Fever-producing substances found in some distilled waters. *American Journal of Physiology* **67**, 90–104.

Seibert F. B. (1925) The cause of many febrile reactions following intravenous injections. *American Journal of Physiology* **71**, 621–651.

Seibert F. B. and Bourn J. M. (1925) The cause of many febrile reactions following intravenous injections II. The bacteriology of twelve distilled waters. *American Journal of Physiology* **71**, 652–659.

Seibert F. B. and Mendel L. B. (1923) Protein fevers. *American Journal of Physiology* **67**, 105–110.

Simon S., Tóth M., Wallerstein G. and Remény Z. (1976) Studies with the international pyrogen standard on the sensitivity and reproducibility of pharmacopoeial pyrogen testing. *Journal of Pharmacy and Pharmacology* **28**, 111–116.

Simon S., Tóth M., Wallerstein, G. and Remény Z. (1977) Studies on the sensitivity and reproducibility of pharmacopoeial pyrogen testing. *Developments in Biological Standardization* **34**, 75–84.

Stammati A. P., Silano V. and Zucco F. (1981) Toxicology investigations with cell culture systems. *Toxicology* **20**, 91–153.

Tsuji K., Steindler K. A. and Harrison S. J. (1980) Limulus Amebocyte Lysate assay for detection and quantitation of endotoxin in a small-volume parenteral product. *Applied and Environmental Microbiology* **40**, 533–538.

U. S. Department of Health and Human Services (1987) Guideline on validation of the Limulus Amebocyte Lysate test as an end-product endotoxin test for human and animal parenteral drugs, biological products and medical devices. U. S. D. H. S. S. December, 1987.

Van Dijk P. and Van de Voorde H. (1977) Factors affecting pyrogen testing in rabbits. *Developments in Biological Standardization* **34**, 57–63.

Van Noordwijk J. (1979) A comparison between the Limulus Amebocyte Lysate test and the rabbit pyrogen test. *Journal de Pharmacie Belgique* **34**, 142–144.

Wachtel R. E. and Tsuji K. (1977) Comparison of Limulus amebocyte lysates and the correlation with the United States Pharmacopeial Pyrogen Test. *Applied and Environmental Microbiology* **33**, 1265–1269.

Walum E. and Peterson A. (1983) Acute toxicity testing in cultures of mouse neuroblastoma cells. *Acta Pharmacologica et Toxicologica* **52**, 100–114.

Walum E. and Peterson A. (1984) On the application of cultured neuroblastoma cells in chemical toxicity screening. *Journal of Toxicology and Environmental Health* **13**, 511–520.

Wardle E. N. (1975) Endotoxin and acute renal failure. *Nephron* **14**, 321–332.

Weary M. E., Donohue G., Pearson F. C. and Story K. (1980) Relative potencies of four reference endotoxin standards as measured by the Limulus Amebocyte Lysate and USP rabbit pyrogenicity tests. *Applied and Environmental Microbiology* **40**, 1148–1151.

Weary M. E., Pearson F. C., Bohon J. and Donohue G. (1982) The activity of various endotoxins in the USP rabbit test and in three different LAL tests. *Progress in Clinical and Biological Research* **93**, 365–379.

Weary M. E. and Wallin R. F. (1973) The rabbit pyrogen test. *Laboratory Animal Science* **23**, 677–681.

Weidner P., Müller-Calgan H., and Ebert A. (1987) NP-1: A liquid endotoxin standard. *Progress in Clinical and Biological Research* **231**, 115–131.

Weiss P.J. (1978) Pyrogen testing. *Journal of the Parenteral Drug Association* **32,** 236–241.
Wright S.D. (1991) Multiple receptors for endotoxin. *Current Opinion in Immunology* **3,** 83–90.
Zanetti C., De Angelis I., Stammati A.-M. and Zucco F. (1992) Evaluation of toxicity testing of 20 MEIC chemicals on Hep-2 cells using two viability endpoints. *ATLA* **20,** 120–125.
Zucco F. (1992) In vitro test validation: No room for conflict with "mechanistic" studies. *ATLA* **20,** 565–566.

5 The Fund for the Replacement of Animals in Medical Experiments (FRAME): 23 Years of Campaigning for the Three Rs

Michael Balls and Julia H. Fentem

Summary

The Fund for the Replacement of Animals in Medical Experiments (FRAME) was established in 1969, to work to relieve the suffering of animals used as subjects in biomedical research, and to promote and support research into acceptable new techniques as substitutes for the use of animals in all such research. FRAME's contributions to progress based on the Three Rs (replacement, refinement, reduction) concept of alternatives are reviewed, with particular emphasis on FRAME's journal *ATLA (Alternatives to Laboratory Animals)*, the work of the FRAME Toxicity Committee, the FRAME Research Programme, the British Animals (Scientific Procedures) Act 1986 and Directive 86/609/EEC, the use of non-human primates as laboratory animals, and the validation and regulatory acceptance of relevant and reliable non-animal toxicity tests and testing strategies. Finally, FRAME's plans for the immediate future and longer-term expectations are outlined.

Abbreviations. ATLA = Alternatives to Laboratory Animals; BVA = British Veterinary Association; COLIPA = Comité de Liaison des Associations Européennes de l'Industrie de la Parfumerie, des Produits Cosmétiques et de Toilette; CRAE = Committee for the Reform of Animal Experimentation; CTPA = Cosmetic, Toiletry & Perfumery Association.

5.1 Introduction: The early years

The Fund for the Replacement of Animals in Medical Experiments (FRAME) was officially established as a charitable trust in England in 1969, with the following aims (Anon., 1969):

- To promote the mental and moral improvement of mankind by working to relieve suffering and cruelty to animals, particularly when such animals are being used as subjects for medical, biological, pharmaceutical and other associated researches.
- To promote, or assist in the provision of, research into acceptable new techniques and substitutes for the use of animals in such medical, biological, pharmaceutical and associated researches, and in the publication of the results of all such research.

Alternatives to Animal Testing. New Ways in the Biomedical Sciences, Trends and Progress.
Reinhardt, C. A. (ed.). 1994. © VCH, Weinheim.

To further these objectives, the honorary trustees of FRAME (who must number a minimum of four and a maximum of six) were empowered (Anon., 1969) to:

– Give all possible encouragement, advice, information and assistance to those engaged in the fields of medical, biological, pharmaceutical and associated researches involving experiments on animals, so as to avoid unintentional cruelty and unnecessary suffering.
– Further human ingenuity toward expanding existing techniques for replacing animals in such experimentation and toward discovering more-reliable, humane and ethical methods of experimentation.
– Provide or assist in providing appropriate equipment and financial aid to existing and/or new laboratories.
– Stimulate the revision of medical and biological educational curricula, so that full regard is paid to acceptable and efficient substitutes for animals in experimentation and so that the use of sentient living animals in research and routine testing in medicine and biology is reduced as far as possible.

The setting-up of FRAME by its founding trustees, under the chairmanship of Mrs. Dorothy Hegarty, was one of the most important initiatives, and certainly one of the most long-lasting and influential, to follow the publication, in 1959, of Russell and Burch's book, *The Principles of Humane Experimental Technique* (Russell and Burch, 1959).

Russell and Burch classified humane techniques under the headings of *Replacement*, *Reduction* and *Refinement*, now known as the *Three Rs*. One of FRAME's most important contributions has been the promotion of a Three Rs definition of *alternatives*, based on that of Professor David Smyth (1978), for which FRAME was awarded the first Marchig Animal Welfare Award of the World Society for the Protection of Animals in 1980: *Alternatives are any procedures which can completely replace the need for animal experiments, reduce the number of animals required, or diminish the amount of pain or distress suffered by animals in meeting the essential needs of man and other animals.*

In its early days, FRAME was run from a spare room in Mrs. Hegarty's house in Wool Road, Wimbledon, a London suburb also famous for its tennis tournament. In 1971, an office was opened nearby, in a former shop at 312a Worple Road, Raynes Park. Much effort was devoted to establishing FRAME as a world information and bibliography center devoted to more-humane methods of research. In addition, contacts were made with many scientists, politicians and industrialists, who welcomed this active promotion of a middle way. As Dr. Bernard Dixon, then editor of *The New Scientist* put it, FRAME is "the scientists' own ginger group" and is providing "a valuable service in changing the climate of thought." FRAME's activities were also characterized by a realism which was not particularly welcomed by the more antivivisection-minded, and Mrs. Hegarty was forced to write in April 1973 (Hegarty, 1973):

We are all anxious to see animals replaced in medical experiments whenever and as speedily as possible. It must, however, be realised that animal experimentation has become so firmly entrenched that changes will only be effected by careful thought and planning, and not by hurried and impetuous demands made without due consideration.

We still have to make similar statements several times each month – in reply to enquirers who have been misled by the rather simplistic literature of certain other organizations.

A number of significant events took place during the 1970s, within and outside FRAME, which contributed to the "changing climate" referred to by Dr. Dixon. For example, the news that more than 5.6 million experiments on living vertebrates had been started in Great Britain in 1971, led to a strong public reaction, which was later to be refuelled by the news that ICI were using beagles to develop a "safe" smoking material and by the publication of Richard Ryder's book, *Victims of Science* (Ryder, 1975).

Meanwhile, 1976 was declared Animal Welfare Year, to mark the centenary of the passing of the Cruelty to Animals Act 1876, and the British government indicated its willingness to consider reforming the legislation which controlled animal experimentation. Also in 1976, Dr. Andrew Rowan became the trust's senior scientist. He greatly increased FRAME's contacts with scientists and provided various authoritative position papers, e. g. on the use of non-human primates in polio vaccine production and testing, and on the LD_{50} test. Another of Rowan's main contributions was the organization of a highly successful conference on The Use of Alternatives in Drug Research, held at the Royal Society in London in 1978 (Rowan and Stratmann, 1980).

A number of other particularly significant developments, which were to lead to the emergence of FRAME as it is known today, took place during the period 1979–81. The Founders of FRAME retired and handed over to a new generation of trustees, the FRAME Toxicity Committee and the FRAME Research Programme were set up, a Parliamentary Group was established, and a Triple Alliance of the British Veterinary Association (BVA), the Committee for the Reform of Animal Experimentation (CRAE) and FRAME was formed, with the intention of making specific proposals to the government concerning the reform of the 1876 Act. Most significant of all, however, was the decision that FRAME should move from London to Nottingham, so that an active collaboration could be developed with the University of Nottingham and, in particular, with its Medical School.

The growth of FRAME in its first 23 years is perhaps best illustrated by its expenditure. Early on, the charity benefited from the generosity of Lady Kinnoull's Sylvanus Trust, but, even by 1973, annual expenditure was running at only about £6500. In 1982, the trustees said that £40 000 would be needed to sustain the activities planned for the year ahead, and our budget for 1992–93 was £760 000.

FRAME's main activities and achievements will be summarized in the following pages, and we will conclude this brief review with some thoughts about the trust's future plans and expectations.

5.2   Publications

In the search for its goal of becoming a world information center on replacement alternatives, FRAME launched a journal in 1973, entitled *Abstracts of Alternatives to Laboratory Animals*. Reviewers were appointed to survey the biomedical literature and provide summaries of papers involving the use of non-animal methods. The journal became *ATLA Abstracts* in 1974, then, in 1981, some three or four years after Rowan had begun to include review articles, the journal was relaunched as *ATLA (Alternatives to Laboratory Animals)*. *ATLA* was still produced from camera-ready typescript, but now contained editorials, news and views, comments, review articles and book reviews, and the original abstracts were retained only as "selected titles."

In 1983, *ATLA* was further redesigned and became a quarterly, single-column, type-set journal with a distinguished international editorial board. 1990 saw a further redesign and a change to a two-column format, when volume 18 was published as a 368-page, single-issue volume, partly to celebrate FRAME's twenty-first anniversary, and partly to ensure that publication years would in future coincide with calendar years.

ATLA now has a managing editor and three regional editors (for the U. K. and the rest of the world, Europe, and North America). Its editorial board is representative of ten countries, and the journal is now distributed to 48 countries. The journal regularly publishes short papers based on the meetings of a number of national and regional organizations, including the Scandinavian Society for Cell Toxicology, the French Societé de Pharmacotoxicologie Cellulaire, the Italian Group for the Application of Tissue Culture in Toxicology (now CELL-TOX, the Assozione Italia de Tossicologia *In Vitro*), and the Dutch Toxicology *In Vitro* Group.

Over the years, *ATLA* has contained many important editorials, but none more so than those published in 1992, which have stimulated a lively, and as yet unfinished, debate on the use of correlative and mechanistic in vitro tests (Balls, 1992a; Balls and Fentem, 1992; Flint, 1992; Green, 1992; Walum, 1992). Another memorable issue contained ten review articles (Balls *et al.*, 1987), on the U. S. Congress Office of Technology Assessment Report on *Alternatives to Animal Use in Research, Education and Testing* (Anon., 1986).

The reputation of *ATLA* is perhaps best summarized by the following comment by Dr. Francis Roe, concerning Volume 18 (Roe, 1991):

> From the start, *ATLA* ... has provided a forum for continuing debate on how to reduce the use of animals. Articles from those who object to the use of animals for establishing the safety of, e. g. ingredients in cosmetics, have appeared alongside articles stressing the need to validate the use of *in vitro* procedures, before they are used in place of animal tests. As this debate continues, *ATLA* will remain a hybrid between science and conscience: a high-class toxicological journal with an underlying continuing message. The contents of Volume 18 weigh up the present situation, criticise the stances taken by regulatory bodies, outline possible ways forward, warn against the adoption of unvalidated tests, and promise no quick solutions.

Over the years, FRAME has also published many pamphlets and position papers, plus a series of newsletters for its supporters and other interested parties, beginning with a twice-yearly *Progress Report*, then, from 1979, *FRAME Technical News*. In 1984, these two type-script, camera-ready publications were combined into *FRAME NEWS*, which was typeset and soon became an influential source of information and comment. However, some of FRAME's supporters among the general public found *FRAME NEWS* to be too technical, while some of our scientifically-qualified readers no doubt found it tiresome to be confronted with details of fundraising events, so *Friends of FRAME* began to appear in 1989.

5.3   Education

From its beginning, FRAME has tried to meet all the requests received from schools and colleges, to provide speakers to take part in debates on the animal experimentation issue or to give talks on alternatives. In return, many school students have taken part in fundraising events of various kinds.

Large numbers of enquiries are received from schools, especially now that animal welfare matters are included in various syllabuses, and especially in those leading to post-16 examinations. As a result, a 16-page booklet on *Animal Experiments* has been published with the support of a consortium of cosmetics manufacturers and in collaboration with Hobsons Publishing (Balls *et al.*, 1992). A second booklet, on *Developing Alternatives to Animal Experimentation*, appeared early in 1993 (Fentem *et al.*, 1993). It is also our intention to produce two similar, four-page, pamphlets, which will be sent automatically to all enquirers. We cannot, however, expect to match the resources invested in education by the large antivivisection and pro-animal research organisations.

FRAME is also a partner in an EC TEMPUS project, which involves collaboration with the University of Nottingham, ZEBET, the Free University of Berlin, and Charles University, Hradec Králové, Czech Republic, to promote the Three Rs concept and to provide training in non-animal methods in the former socialist countries of central and eastern Europe (see Červinka *et al.*, 1994, this volume).

5.4   The FRAME Toxicity Committee

In 1978, FRAME decided to set up an expert committee, consisting of toxicologists, pharmacologists and other scientists from relevant disciplines, to review toxicity testing procedures, and to assess the prospects for developing non-animal systems to replace studies on living animals. The FRAME Toxicity Committee began to meet in 1979, and produced its first report in 1982 (Anon., 1982). The Committee made 30 specific recommendations, which were discussed at a conference held at the Royal Society, the proceedings of which were subsequently published (Balls *et al.*, 1983).

The Committee was re-formed in 1989 and produced a second report in 1990, which contained 66 conclusions and recommendations (Anon., 1991). Again, a conference was held to discuss the report, this time at the Royal College of Physicians in London, the proceedings of which were subsequently published (Balls *et al.*, 1991). The Committee now proposes to take steps to promote the implementation of the recommendations of its 14 working parties.

5.5   Legislation

The BVA/CRAE/FRAME Alliance began to meet in 1981, and a set of proposals for reform of the Cruelty to Animals Act 1876 were sent to the Home Secretary in March 1983 (Anon., 1983a). Two months later, the British government produced its own proposals in a White Paper (Anon., 1983b), which bore a remarkable resemblance to those of BVA/CRAE/FRAME.

From that moment, members of the Triple Alliance had regular meetings with government ministers and civil servants at the Home Office, and acted as advisers at all stages of the preparation of what was to become the Animals (Scientific Procedures) Act 1986. Along the way, the government produced a second White Paper (Anon., 1985), which contained the following remarkable Three Rs statement: "All experiments which are unnecessary, use unnecessarily large numbers of animals, or are unnecessarily painful, are indefensible."

The members of the Triple Alliance were instrumental in seeing that a number of provisions were included in the Act, including the following two important clauses:

> In determining whether and on what terms to grant a project licence the Secretary of State shall weigh the likely adverse effects on the animals concerned against the benefit likely to accrue as a result of the program to be specified in the licence; *and*
> The Secretary of State shall not grant a project licence unless he is satisfied that the applicant has given adequate consideration to the feasibility of achieving the purpose of the program to be specified in the licence by means not involving the use of protected animals.

During this period, the chairman of the FRAME trustees was invited to join the Advisory Committee which advised the Home Secretary on the operation of the 1876 Act, and then the new Animal Procedures Committee, established by the 1986 Act.

EC Directive 86/609 was published in 1986, and was based on a Convention of the Council of Europe, published earlier that year. FRAME has a contract to advise the Commission of the EC on the implementation of the Directive, and has produced a number of commissioned reports on specific topics related to animal experimentation and the alternatives.

FRAME has also been invited to advise many other official bodies, including the Council of International Organizations in the Medical Sciences (CIOMS), during the preparation of its guiding principles on biomedical research involving animals, the U. S. Office of Technology Assessment (OTA), and the British Parliamentary Office of Science and Technology (POST).

5.6   The use of non-human primates as laboratory animals

FRAME has long been concerned about the use of non-human primates in laboratories, partly because, unless standards of care of these highly-sentient animals are very high, and unless controls on their use are very stringent, it is unlikely that other laboratory animals will fare very well.

On 2 January 1987, on the day when the Animals (Scientific Procedures) Act 1986 came into force, FRAME and CRAE presented the Home Secretary with a report on non-human primate use, which contained 17 specific suggestions (Anon., 1987a). Such was the esteem in which FRAME and CRAE were held, one of the proposals (that "primates" be subdivided into a number of groups in the annual Home Office statistics of animal use) was even put into force before the report was officially delivered and published. The Home Secretary subsequently accepted all but one of the other proposals (Anon., 1987b).

Subsequently, a survey on published research which had been undertaken before the new law came into effect, was conducted for the Royal Society for the Prevention of Cruelty to Animals (RSPCA) and FRAME (Hampson *et al.*, 1990). Many causes of concern were identified. As a result of this report and of subsequent events, the Animal Procedures Com-

mittee is currently conducting a review of how the 1986 Act is being applied to the use of non-human primates.

FRAME has also been involved in various campaigns to improve the care of chimpanzees used in laboratories in Europe and the U. S. A. (they have not been used in Great Britain for many years), and to prevent, on scientific, as well as animal welfare, grounds, any significant increase in their use in AIDS research (Anon., 1988a, 1988b).

5.7   The FRAME Research Programme

At about the time that FRAME moved to Nottingham, it was decided that a research program on alternatives should be set up. Early in 1982, four laboratories were invited to take part in a collaborative study with the aim of developing a cytotoxicity test for basal/intrinsic toxicity. The laboratories were located at the University of Nottingham Medical School, St George's Hospital Medical School, London, the Robens Institute at the University of Surrey, and Huntingdon Research Center. Selected industrial companies were invited to provide financial support, and the £180 000 required for a three-year program was raised within a few months. The first phase of the program led to the development of the FRAME kenacid blue method and to the setting up of the first interlaboratory toxicity test validation scheme outside the field of genotoxicity (Knox *et al.*, 1986).

In 1984, the British government awarded FRAME £160 000 over a three-year period – the first such grant given in Britain specifically for alternatives research. It would be hard to overestimate the value of this award in terms of the raising of FRAME's credibility.

The FRAME Research Programme is now about to enter its fourth phase, and nearly £2 million has so far been spent on alternatives research. Research is now being carried out at Nottingham, Surrey and Huntingdon, and at the University of Hertfordshire. The topics under investigation include neurotoxicology, hepatotoxicology, nephrotoxicology, immuno-toxicology, irritancy, and carcinogenicity. This research is currently being supported by Avon Cosmetics Limited, Boots The Chemist Limited, Bristol-Myers Squibb Company, Elida Gibbs Limited, Fisons Pharmaceuticals, Gillette U. K. Limited, Glaxo Group Research, Hoechst U. K. Limited, Huntingdon Research Center Limited, Johnson & Johnson Limited, Marks and Spencer plc, Millipore Corporation, L'Oréal, Pfizer Limited, Reckitt & Colman plc, Rhône-Poulenc Limited, Rimmel International Limited, J Sainsbury plc, Sensiq Cosmetics, SmithKline Beecham, Superdrug Stores plc, Tesco Stores Limited, and Unilever Research. In addition, in recent years, significant support has also been received from the EC for international collaborative studies, as well as from the British government. Collaborative studies are now in progress with other laboratories in the Czech Republic, France, Germany, Poland, and the U. S. A., as well as in Britain. Up to the end of 1992, 96 publications had resulted from the research conducted as part of the FRAME Research Program.

5.8   Other collaborations

In addition to the collaborative arrangements already mentioned, FRAME has provided the Secretariat for ERGATT (European Research Group for Alternatives in Toxicity Testing), a group of individuals based in eight European countries, who are committed to maximizing the potential of in vitro toxicology.

ERGATT members have been involved in two major workshops on the principles of validation and regulatory acceptance of non-animal toxicity tests (see below) and, most recently, in setting up ECITTS (the ERGATT/CFN Integrated *In Vitro* Toxicity Testing Scheme; Walum *et al.*, 1992).

With the support of the Commission of the EC, FRAME and ERGATT have established INVITTOX, a unique in vitro toxicology databank, which provides interested scientists with up-to-date details of how in vitro tests should be performed (Ungar, 1992).

The relationship which has developed between FRAME and the University of Nottingham has been particularly important to FRAME's development since the move to Nottingham took place in 1981. Alternatives research has been conducted in the Departments of Human Morphology, Physiology & Pharmacology, and Biochemistry. With the support of donations given to the FRAME Anniversary Appeal, the FRAME Alternatives Laboratory has been rebuilt and equipped in the Department of Human Morphology. Many of FRAME's young scientists have conducted part-time research at the University, for which they have been awarded PhDs.

5.9   Validation and acceptance

FRAME has been closely involved in discussions on the principles of the process of validation, whereby the relevance and reproducibility of non-animal methods are evaluated. A workshop on validation, organized with ERGATT and the Center for Alternatives to Animal Testing at Johns Hopkins University, Baltimore, U. S. A., took place early in 1990 (Balls *et al.*, 1990a).

The FRAME research groups have taken part in a number of validation studies organized on behalf of the U. S. Soap & Detergent Association, the U. S. Cosmetic, Toiletry & Fragrance Association, and the EC, as well as in a number of validation studies with companies. We are currently involved in two international studies, partly supported by the EC, on the use of cytotoxicity tests in predicting the acute lethal potencies of chemicals, and on the evaluation of potential alternatives to the Draize eye test. The latter study will cost £1.4 million, and involves 9 tests, 60 chemicals, and 36 laboratories based in 9 countries (7 in Europe, plus the U. S. A. and Japan).

No less important than validation is the question of how methods and combinations of methods which emerge successfully from a validation study, can be made acceptable to the national and international authorities responsible for controlling the use of new chemicals and products of many kinds, and for approving the methods used in predicting their potential toxicity and assessing their safety in various circumstances. A workshop on acceptance, organized by ERGATT and financially supported by the EC, was held in 1990 (Balls *et al.*, 1990b).

Validation and acceptance will be major topics of interest and concern thoughout the 1990s (Balls, 1992a, 1992b; Balls and Fentem, 1992; Green, 1992). A European Centre for the Validation of Alternative Methods (ECVAM) has recently been established at the EC's Joint Research Centre, at Ispra in Italy. The chairman of the FRAME trustees has been appointed director of this influential European institution (see Marafante and Balls, 1994, this volume).

5.10 The cosmetics testing issue

In 1977, FRAME produced a leaflet entitled *What Price Vanity?*, which spelled out the case against using animals to test cosmetics ingredients or finished products, and was accompanied by a list of companies which claimed to supply products which had "not been tested on animals."

However, following discussions with various cosmetics companies and, in particular, with the Cosmetic, Toiletry & Perfumery Association (CTPA), the shallowness of this approach was recognized and the leaflet was withdrawn. FRAME then developed its own objective and rational approach to the controversial issue of cosmetics testing. Basically, it is that the safety of cosmetics is no less important than that of any other kind of product which is legitimately made and marketed, and that the way forward is to work actively with companies committed to the development and validation of relevant and reliable replacement alternative tests and testing strategies.

As a result, FRAME has developed a number of research collaborations with cosmetics companies, has been involved in a number of validation studies on alternative methods for cosmetics testing, and has been regularly consulted by the CTPA, COLIPA (the European Federation of Cosmetic Industry Associations), and the EC. An original scheme for assessing the safety of cosmetic ingredients and products manufactured and/or marketed in Europe has been proposed (Balls, 1991a), comments on the use of terms such as "cruelty free" and "not tested on animals" have been published (Balls, 1991b), and a 15-point plan for dealing with the animal experimentation issue was put to the 1991 General Assembly of COLIPA (Balls, 1992c). A major review of the issue of cosmetics testing and safety assessment was presented as the 1992 Medal Lecture of the Society of Cosmetic Scientists (Balls, 1992d).

FRAME has also been active in advising various interested parties during the passage of a Sixth Amendment to the EEC Cosmetics Directive (76/768/EEC), an issue which has received regular coverage in *FRAME NEWS*. FRAME believes that reform of the membership and terms of reference of the Scientific Committee on Cosmetology, which advises the EC Commission and the Council of Ministers on matters related to the safety of cosmetics, is essential.

5.11 FRAME and the future

Ever since the first discussions about the foundation of FRAME took place in the years leading up to the signing of the Trust Deed in September 1969, all connected with FRAME, past and present, have done their utmost to promote the aims of the charity and to meet the expectations of its supporters. Nevertheless, while there has been a significant reduction in animal experimentation in Britain, for scientific and economic reasons, as well as in the interests of animal welfare, and while the Three Rs concept is now widely recognized, there is still great scope for eliminating unnecessary animal procedures, for improving the quality of any necessary studies, and for a stronger commitment by scientists and governments to actively seek replacement alternatives. Thus, however successful we may claim to have been up to now, we must strive to be much more effective in the future.

FRAME is now at a crossroads, and some significant new developments are planned for the immediate future. These will include the appointment of new trustees, a greater emphasis on *refinement* without reducing our commitment to *replacement*, an increase in the scale of our research at the University of Nottingham Medical School, the elucidation of proposals on the assessment and weighing of benefit and suffering in animal experimentation, the development of a strategy on the integrated use of in vitro methods and computer predictions in toxicity evaluation, the production of a position paper outlining ways of reducing experimental procedures conducted on dogs and cats (while continuing our efforts on behalf of non-human primates, on the grounds that animals of these three types, on their own initiative, form special bonds with human beings, and therefore should not be used as laboratory animals), and an investigation into the ethical and scientific issues raised by genetic engineering in animals.

FRAME has two overriding goals for the 1990s. The first is to play an active part in securing the acceptance of one or more non-animal tests and/or testing strategies as *total* replacements for the use of conventional animal tests in assessing the toxic potential of chemicals and products. The second is to work toward the day when, instead of having to justify the search for non-animal methods in a world where animal experimentation is the norm in so many fundamental and applied biomedical investigations, we will be able to transfer the burden of justification to others, who will themselves have to argue convincingly that the continued use of animals is scientifically necessary, and therefore ethically acceptable, in a diminishing number of highly-specific circumstances.

References

Anonymous (1969) *Trust Deed Constituting the Fund for the Replacement of Animals in Medical Experiments.* FRAME, London.
Anonymous (1982) Report of the FRAME Toxicity Committee. *ATLA* **10,** 4–43.
Anonymous (1983a) *Animal Experimentation in the United Kingdom: Proposals Submitted to the Home Secretary jointly by the BVA, CRAE and FRAME.* 8 pp. CRAE, Edinburgh.
Anonymous (1983b) *Scientific Procedures on Living Animals* (Cmnd 8883). 34 pp. HMSO, London.
Anonymous (1985) *Scientific Procedures on Living Animals* (Cmnd 9521). 25 pp. HMSO, London.
Anonymous (1986) *Alternatives to Animal Use in Research, Testing and Education.* U. S. Congress, Office of Technology Assessment, Washington DC.
Anonymous (1987a) *The Use of Non-human Primates as Laboratory Animals in Great Britain.* 20 pp. FRAME/CRAE, Nottingham.
Anonymous (1987b) Response of the British Home Secretary to the FRAME/CRAE report on The Use of Non-human Primates as Laboratory Animals in Great Britain. *ATLA* **15,** 141–146.
Anonymous (1988a) Pressure for better care for chimpanzees in captivity. *ATLA* **15,** 255–259.
Anonymous (1988b) Chimpanzees and the fight against AIDS. *FRAME NEWS* **18,** 3–5.
Anonymous (1991) Animals and alternatives in toxicology: Present status and future prospects (The Second Report of the FRAME Toxicity Committee). *ATLA* **19,** 116–138.
Balls M. (1991a) On establishing the safety of cosmetic ingredients and products produced and/or marketed within the European Economic Community. *ATLA* **19,** 237–244.
Balls M. (1991b) Comments on labelling related to the animal testing of cosmetic ingredients and products manufactured and/or marketed within the European Economic Community. *ATLA* **19,** 302–307.
Balls M. (1992a) *In vitro* test validation: high-hurdling, but *not* pole vaulting. *ATLA* **20,** 355–357.
Balls M. (1992b) The validation and acceptance of *in vitro* toxicity tests. In *In Vitro Methods In Toxicology.* Edited by G. Jolles and A. Cordier. pp. 511–519. Academic Press Ltd., London.
Balls M. (1992c) What should the cosmetic industry do about the animal testing controversy? *International Journal of Cosmetic Science* **14,** 1–9.
Balls M. (1992d) For beauty lives with kindness – some thoughts on cosmetics testing and safety assessment. *International Journal of Cosmetic Science* **14,** 199–227.

Balls M., Blaauboer B., Brusick D., Frazier J., Lamb D., Pemberton M., Reinhardt C., Roberfroid M., Rosenkranz H., Schmid B., Spielmann H., Stammati A.-L. and Walum E. (1990a) Report and recommendations of the CAAT/ERGATT workshop on the validation of toxicity test procedures. *ATLA* **18,** 313–337.

Balls M., Botham P., Cordier A., Fumero S., Kayser D., Koëter H., Koundakjian P., Gunnar Lindquist N., Meyer O., Pioda L., Reinhardt C., Rozemond H., Smyrniotis T., Spielmann H., Van Looy H., van der Venne M. T. and Walum, E. (1990b) Report and recommendations of an international workshop on promotion of the regulatory acceptance of validated non-animal toxicity test procedures. *ATLA* **18,** 339–344.

Balls M., Bridges J. and Southee J. (Editors) (1991) *Animals and Alternatives in Toxicology. Present Status and Future Prospects.* Macmillan Press, Basingstoke, and VCH Publishers, New York.

Balls M. and Fentem J. H. (1992) The use of basal cytotoxicity and target organ toxicity tests in hazard identification and risk assessment. *ATLA* **20,** 368–388.

Balls M., Fentem J. and Joint E. (1992) *Animal Experiments. A resource book for A-level General Studies and 16–19 Entitlement Curriculum.* 16 pp. Hobsons Publishing plc, Cambridge.

Balls M., Riddell R. J. and Worden A. N. (Editors) (1983) *Animals and Alternatives in Toxicity Testing.* Academic Press, London, New York.

Balls M., Sprigge T. L. S., Drewett R. F., Benford D. J., Heywood R., Morton D. B., Bawden D., McCormick H., Hollands C. and Haywood S. (1987) The US Congress Office of Technology Assessment Report on *Alternatives to Animal Use in Research, Testing and Education. ATLA* **14,** 289–374.

Červinka M., Červinková Z., Balls M. and Spielmann H. (1994) Alternatives to experiments with animals in medical education: A TEMPUS Joint European Project. In *Alternatives to Animal Testing. New Ways in the Biomedical Sciences, Trends and Progress.* Edited by C. A. Reinhardt. pp. 119–123. VCH Verlagsgesellschaft, Weinheim.

Fentem J., Balls M. and Robinson P. (1993) *Developing Alternatives to Animal Experimentation.* 20 pp. Hobsons Publishing plc, Cambridge.

Flint O. P. (1992) *In vitro* test validation: a house built on sand. *ATLA* **20,** 196–198.

Green S. (1992) *In vitro* test validation and regulatory animal testing: a house built on sand versus a house of cards? *ATLA* **20,** 567–570.

Hampson J., Southee J., Howell D. and Balls M. (1990) An RSPCA/FRAME survey on the use of non-human primates as laboratory animals in Great Britain, 1984–1988. *ATLA* **17,** 335–400.

Hegarty D. (1973) In conclusion. *FRAME Progress Report* **7,** 3.

Knox P., Uphill P. F., Fry J. R., Benford D. J. and Balls M. (1986) The FRAME multi-center project on *in vitro* cytotoxicology. *Food and Chemical Toxicology* **24,** 457–463.

Marafante E. and Balls M. (1994) The European Centre for the Validation of Alternative Methods (ECVAM). In *Alternatives to Animal Testing. New Ways in the Biomedical Sciences, Trends and Progress.* Edited by C. A. Reinhardt. pp. 21–25. VCH Verlagsgesellschaft, Weinheim.

Roe F. J. C. (1991) [Review of *Alternatives to Laboratory Animals,* Volume 18]. *Human and Experimental Toxicology* **10,** 296.

Rowan A. N. and Stratmann C. J. (1980) *The Use of Alternatives in Drug Research.* Macmillan Press Ltd., London.

Russell W. M. S. and Burch R. L. (1959) *The Principles of Humane Experimental Technique.* Methuen & Co. Ltd., London.

Ryder R. D. (1975) *Victims of Science.* Davis-Poynter Ltd., London.

Smyth D. H. (1978) *Alternatives to Animal Experiments.* Scolar Press, London.

Ungar K. (1992) The INVITTOX data bank of *in vitro* techniques in toxicology. *Human and Experimental Toxicology* **11,** 151–154.

Walum E. (1992) *In vitro* test validation: should it obey laws, recognise uncertainty principles or follow scientific practices? *ATLA* **20,** 502–503.

Walum E., Balls M., Bianchi V., Blaauboer B., Bolcsfoldi G., Guillouzo A., Moore G. A., Odland L., Reinhardt C. and Spielmann H. (1992) ECITTS: an integrated approach to the application of *in vitro* test systems to the hazard assessment of chemicals. *ATLA* **20,** 406–428.

6 Animal Use and Alternatives: Developments in the Netherlands

L. F. M. van Zutphen

Summary

Recent developments are described which have contributed to the reduction of animal use, to the welfare of experimental animals, and to the quality of animal experiments. Legislation has been the main impetus behind most of these developments. The developments described here are the establishment of: a) the Platform for Alternatives to Animal Experiments (1987), which has a budget of 1.5 million guilders per year for funding the search for alternatives; b) a national center for alternatives, expected to be operational by 1994; c) institutional animal experimentation committees with the task of advising on the admissibility of experiments based upon balancing the benefit of the experiment against the suffering of the animals; d) training programs, which have been made compulsory by law for persons who are involved in animal experimentation; and e) the information center (PREX) at the Department of Laboratory Animal Science, Utrecht, with computerized databases on several aspects of animal use and alternatives. These activities support the general policy of most institutions which have a license for animal experimentation, which is to reduce animal use and to introduce alternatives wherever feasible.

Abbreviations. AEC = animal experimentation committee; NCA = Netherlands Centre for Alternatives to Animal Experiments; PREX = Proefdierkundig Expertisecentrum.

6.1 Introduction

Approximately one million vertebrate animals were used for research, education, and testing in the Netherlands in 1990 (VHI, 1991). Approximately 80% of these animals are rodents. During the past five years, the overall use has decreased by about 20%. Figure 6-1 shows the various purposes for which the animals are used.

The use of animals can be further subdivided according to the degree of suffering they experience when exposed to experimental procedures. Three (arbitrary) categories have been determined:

– minor animal suffering (e.g. observing animals in behavioral studies, single blood sampling, immunization without adjuvants);

Alternatives to Animal Testing. New Ways in the Biomedical Sciences, Trends and Progress.
Reinhardt, C. A. (ed.). 1994. © VCH, Weinheim.

USE OF ANIMALS IN RESEARCH AND EDUCATION

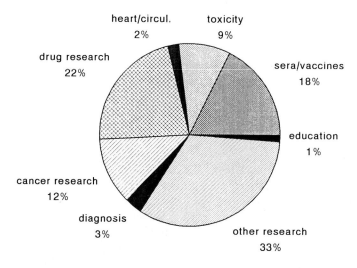

Figure 6-1. Distribution of animal use for research purposes (including testing) and education in The Netherlands. The total number of vertebrate animals is about 1 million (source: VHI, 1991).

– moderate animal suffering (e. g. repeated blood sampling, recovery from general anesthesia);
– severe animal suffering (e. g. LD_{50} test, starvation, vaccine potency tests).

When adhering to this categorization, the 1990 statistics on animal use reveal that the degree of suffering is minor or non-existent in approximately 53 % of the animals, moderate for approximately 23 % and severe for approximately 24 % (see Figure 6-2).

It is now generally accepted that the replacement of animal use, though important, is not the only objective when searching for alternatives to animal experimentation. Every method or procedure that contributes to a reduction of animal use or to a decrease in animal suffering may also be considered as an alternative (Hendriksen and Koëter, 1991).

This paper outlines some of the developments that have taken place in the Netherlands which are in line with this concept of alternatives.

6.2   Legislation

As with most laws regarding the protection of animals used for scientific purposes, the Dutch law on animal experimentation (Experiments on Animals Act, 1977) contains several provisions which contribute to the concept of alternatives as described above (van Zutphen *et al.*, 1989):

– It is not permissible to use an animal for a purpose that could equally be achieved by in-vitro methods, or other procedures which do not require the use of animals.

ANIMAL USE IN BIOMEDICAL RESEARCH
(degree of suffering)

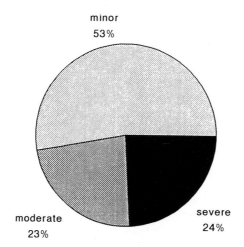

Figure 6-2. Diagram illustrating the subdivision of animal use according to the degree of suffering. See text for explanation of the categories of discomfort (source: VHI, 1991).

– The use of anesthetics or analgesics is mandatory where appreciable pain is anticipated and may only be omitted where their use would jeopardize the purpose of the experiment.
– Particular emphasis is put upon the competence and correct attitude of the persons involved in animal experimentation. Education in the field of laboratory animal science, including ethics and alternatives is mandatory.

The 1977 act is presently under revision. One of the proposed changes involves the provision that research protocols must be screened by an animal experimentation committee (AEC). A further provision is to be included which states that where there is a choice, animals with the lowest degree of neurophysiological sensitivity must be selected. These latter provisions have been included in order to bring the Dutch law into line with the EEC Council Directive (EEC, 1986).

6.2   Platform for Alternatives

In 1987 the government established the Platform for Alternatives to Animal Experiments (Platform). This committee comprises representatives from several ministries, the pharmaceutical industry, and animal protection organizations. The task of the Platform is to stimulate the development and introduction of alternatives to animal experiments, to coordinate activities in the field of alternatives at the national level, and to advise the government on the funding of specific projects. Grant applications made by scientists from universities and other research institutions are screened by members of the Platform in order to ascertain whether the proposed objective of the research project is in line with the goals of the Platform.

The projects that do meet with the criteria are sent for further review to a scientific advisory committee. Given the available budget (1.5 million guilders), only a limited number of proposals can be accepted. Nonetheless, the impact of this fund is felt not only because of the direct results which can be achieved by the approved projects, but also because it has a positive influence upon the scientist's appreciation of research specifically dedicated to alternatives. In 1991, approximately 30 projects were supported by funds from the Platform. The money does not go soley to research projects, but also to the production of interactive computer programs and videos, which serve as alternatives to the use of animals in teaching. Included here would be programs on the anesthesiology of the rat, cannulation methods, and the regulation of blood pressure. The use of alternatives in education may also indirectly affect the attitudes of students towards animals.

6.3   A national center for alternatives to animal experiments

The Platform has recently decided to establish the Netherlands Centre for Alternatives (NCA). The purpose of the Centre is the provision of professional support to the Platform. The major task of the NCA is to collect data and to analyze statistics on animal use in order to enable the Platform to select the most relevant targets for funding. The NCA will also compile a database on established alternatives along with ongoing research in this field. Further, it has a part to play in the coordination of validation studies, preferably in cooperation with the European Centre for the Validation of Alternative Methods (ECVAM, Italy). The NCA should also be used as an information center and a national contact point for local (institutional) centers or for individual scientists working on alternatives. The aim is to establish this center, staffed by two to three scientists with part-time secretarial support, early in 1994 in Utrecht.

Despite the fact that animal use is decreasing and the level of interest for alternatives increasing, the total number of animals used for research and testing purposes is still substantial. The present stage of development of in-vitro techniques or other "replacing" alternatives does not justify the assumption that the current in-vivo tests can be totally replaced in the foreseeable future. It is not realistic to fully rely on these alternatives. Other measures must also be taken to ensure that no more animals are used than are absolutely necessary and that those animals that are still being used are treated as humanely as possible. This requires an ethical evaluation of proposed projects before embarking on the experiments, along with the correct attitude and a high degree of competence of the persons involved in the design and performance of the experiments. Information on the use and care of animals must be readily available for these persons.

6.4   Animal experimentation committees (ethics committees)

In the Netherlands, virtually every institution which has a license for animal experiments also has an animal experimentation committee (AEC) or an ethics committee. As already mentioned, if the proposed revision of the law is accepted by parliament, no experiment with animals will be performed before the project has been evaluated by an AEC. The members of this committee are nominated by the license-holder (e. g. the director of the institution) and have to be approved by the National Advisory Committee on Animal Experimentation. It is proposed in the pending law revision that at least one of the members must not be involved in animal experimentation and that at least one member be a specialist in the field of the care and husbandry of animals. The primary task of the AEC is to weigh the benefit of the experiment against the suffering of the animals. It does, however, also take legal and technical aspects into account when judging the admissibility of any given project. Responsibility for the evaluation of the scientific quality (e. g. methodology, adequacy of the approach, quality of the research team in relation to the proposed protocol, etc.) does not lie with the AEC. Projects must be screened and approved by a scientific committee prior to being submitted to the AEC.

When the AEC has reached a decision, it advises the license-holder, who may overrule the view of the AEC and may even approve a project which has been rejected by the AEC. In such a case, the license-holder is obliged to report this to the National Advisory Committee on Animal Experimentation. In such a situation, the project may not be started until a judgment has been given by this committee. Should this committee also reject the proposed project, then it is forbidden to start the project.

Although the formal procedure seems obvious enough, the major problem still exists of how to balance benefit against suffering. The scientist who is preparing a protocol for submission to the AEC is the first person to consider this problem. Subsequently, members of the AEC have to give their views. In order to provide some guidelines, particularly with regard to the practice of ethical reasoning, short one-day courses specifically devoted to this subject are being organized for members of the AECs. This cannot possibly solve all of the problems, but it should be noted that the procedure of screening by AECs in itself has a positive effect on the humane use of animals in experiments. The researcher, knowing that the project will be evaluated on ethical grounds, is more likely to take this aspect into consideration when designing the experiments. This will ensure that less thoughtful projects are not even submitted.

In addition to its task of screening projects, the AEC also plays an important role in the ethical dialogue on animal experimentation within the institution.

Projects that have been approved by the AEC must be performed with great care and carried out by fully competent personnel. Competence depends mainly upon education and training. An outline of the requirements and educational programs which have been instituted in the Netherlands is given below.

6.5   Education

The requirements for the education and training of persons involved in animal experimentation are laid down in the Experiments on Animals Act (1977) and the Experiments on Animals Decree (1985). Education is the cornerstone for the responsible use of animals in research. There are at least three categories of persons involved which need to be considered:

– the animal caretaker/animal technician,
– the scientist who is responsible for the design of the experiment,
– the animal welfare officer.

6.5.1   Animal caretaker/animal technician

Animal caretakers have to complete a training program lasting a year and a half. This program includes a minimum of:

– 500 hours of laboratory animal science,
– 150 hours of basic education (language, mathematics, etc.),
– 800 hours of practical work (on-the-job training).

For animal technicians the training program takes three years and includes at least:

– 1000 hours of laboratory animal science,
– 300 hours of basic education (language; mathematics, etc.),
– 1600 hours of practical work (on-the-job training).

During both of these vocational training programs, emphasis is placed on "hands-on" learning. Animal caretakers and technicians are key persons affecting an animal's wellbeing. Professional care and handling of the animals, both before and during experiments, is important for both the welfare of the animals and the quality of the experiment. Animals often experience more suffering than is necessary when treated by inexperienced persons. The first training programs were organized more than 30 years ago, and nearly all persons presently working as animal caretakers or animal technicians have taken the appropriate courses. Taking effect in 1995, no one without a certificate will be allowed to take part in the care or handling of laboratory animals.

6.5.2   Scientist

By law (Experiments on Animals Decree, 1985), all "new" scientists who wish to take responsibility for the design and conduct of animal experiments must meet at least two basic requirements:

– They must have completed a graduate training program (a Master's degree or equivalent) in one of the biomedical disciplines (e. g. biology, (veterinary) medicine).
– They must have completed a three-week course in laboratory animal science.

When this provision became compulsory, an exemption was given to scientists who were already involved in animal experimentation.

Although the graduate training in one of the biomedical disciplines is seen as the main basis for competence, the three-week course is seen as a major tool in improving the humane use of the animals as well as for the improvement of animal experiments. Implicit here is that both technical and ethical aspects are part of the training program. Russell and Burch's "replacement, reduction, and refinement" principles provide the guidelines for the course. Main topics covered by the course are:

– biology and husbandry of laboratory animals, including behavior, housing conditions and animal well-being;
– gnotobiology, health monitoring and prevention/recognition of diseases;
– genetic standardization and genetic quality control;

– design of animal experiments and analysis of scientific papers;
– anesthesia, analgesia and experimental techniques;
– alternatives to animal experiments;
– ethical aspects and legislation.

Since 1986 more than 2000 students have taken this course. More than 95 % of the students indicated that even if the course were not compulsory, they would still recommend it for every scientist who is intending to use animals for research. According to the students' judgement, the course not only contributes to a more careful and humane use of animals, but also to the quality of animal experiments. Having taken the course, students seem to be more motivated in seeking alternatives for animal use.

The course is coordinated from the Department of Laboratory Animal Science (Utrecht University). With the support of an EC grant, a multi-author handbook containing the theoretical aspects of the course has been prepared (van Zutphen *et al.*, 1993). Commencing in 1993, an international course on laboratory animal science is being organized each year in Utrecht.

6.5.3   Animal welfare officer

Every institute which has a license for conducting animal experiments must appoint a veterinarian or other competent person who is responsible for overseeing the well-being of the animals used for scientific purposes. These persons usually have several other duties as well. They may be (advisory) members of the AEC, or have responsibilities for stimulating the introduction of alternatives. To attain qualification as an animal welfare officer the veterinarian must have taken a one-year post-graduate training program at the Department of Laboratory Animal Science. The standard program consists of six to eight modules with training periods at different institutes along with a six-month research project. The content of the modules and the research project may be adjusted to the experience and specific needs of the individual student. Certain aspects of the standard program may be omitted if sufficient experience already exists in the given areas.

6.6   Documentation and information (PREX)

In 1991, the Department of Laboratory Animal Science established the documentation and information center PREX. The objective of PREX is to collect, classify and make available information covering all aspects of laboratory animal science, including welfare issues and alternatives. This information is available for students, animal welfare officers, and scientists working with animals and will be accessible on-line via computer networks or modem connections by early 1994. By offering this service, PREX aims to assist in the humane and responsible use of animals. At present, several databases are under development:

– Laboratory animal science "core" journals: Literature references (mainly with summaries) of all papers which have been published in the main journals in the field of laboratory animal science (from the first to the most recent issue) are included. This database now contains references of approximately 10000 papers.
– Biological reference values: This database contains 3500 biological items of data regarding laboratory animals (each with a reference to the source).

- Catalogue of inbred strains: The index of inbred strains developed by M. F. Festing (Carshalton, U. K.) has been made available to PREX for on-line distribution.
- Database of veterinary journals: Contains literature references from a selection of journals in the field of clinical veterinary medicine (approximately 40 000 references).
- Alternatives: A database of literature references on alternatives to animal experiments (approximately 3000 references).
- Catalogue of audiovisuals: This database presents an overview of videos, computer programs, slide/tape programs and other teaching aids, complete with the producer's address (approximately 1500 references).
- Books: This database contains the contents of books (at the level of chapters/subchapters) in the field of laboratory animal science, ethics and alternatives.

All these databases are being continually extended, and other databases will be included in the near future. In addition to these specialized databases, several CD-ROM files (MEDLINE, AGRICOLA) are also on-line available.

A user-interface has been developed which has several options:

- access to the PREX host computer (password);
- downloading/transfer of data to a local PC;
- a "view" option to browse through the downloaded file;
- conversion of data to a format that can be imported into ProCite, Cardbox, or Endnote.

Although PREX has been established to serve as a national center for documentation and information, the final aim is to make these databases available for international networking.

6.7   Conclusions

In the Netherlands, as in many Western countries, the number of animals used for scientific purposes is on the decrease. Developments which have contributed to this decrease include legislation, stimulation of the search for alternatives, ethical evaluation of protocols, and education. Education is of particular importance with regard to this issue. The degree of competence and the attitude towards animals are major determinants for the introduction of alternatives and for the humane treatment of animals in research. It is a commonly held view that animal experiments are only acceptable under very strict conditions. These conditions include:

- approval of the project by an animal experimentation committee;
- persons involved in experiments must be competent (education in laboratory animal science, including ethical aspects, is mandatory);
- discomfort and suffering must be kept to the unavoidable minimum;
- housing, care, and handling of the animals must be monitored by an animal welfare officer;
- serious efforts must be taken to develop and use alternatives.

References

EEC (1986) Council Directive of 24 November 1986 on the approximation of laws, regulations and administrative provisions of the Member States regarding the protection of animals used for experimental and other scientific purposes. *Official Journal of the European Communities* **29,** (L358), 1–29.

Hendriksen C. F. M. and Koëter H. B. W. M. (Editors) (1991) *Animals in Biomedical Research: Replacement, Reduction and Refinement: Present Possibilities and Future Prospects.* Elsevier Science Publishers, Amsterdam.

van Zutphen L. F. M., Baumans V. B and Beynen A. C. (Editors) (1993) *Principles of Laboratory Animal Science: A Contribution to the Humane Use and Care of Animals and to the Quality of Experimental Results.* Elsevier Science Publishers, Amsterdam.

van Zutphen L. F. M., Rozemond H. and Beynen A. C. (Editors) (1989) *Animal Experimentation: Legislation and Education.* Department of Laboratory Animal Science, Utrecht University, Utrecht.

Veterinary Public Health Inspectorate (VHI) (1991) *Zo Doende 1990* (VHI Report). Veterinary Public Health Inspectorate, Rijswijk.

7 The RIVM Center for Alternatives to Animal Testing and the Concept of the Three Rs in the Quality Control of Vaccines

Coenraad F. M. Hendriksen

Summary

Each strategy for reducing and refining the use of animals will be successful only if it includes activities that involve institute management and the individual scientist. At these levels in particular, people have the responsibility for the planning and organization of animal experiments, and their interest in alternatives is of utmost importance. A very effective and direct way to make these groups sensitive to the concept of the Three Rs is the establishment of institute-linked centers for alternatives to animal methods. This paper describes the goals and activities of such a center at the National Institute of Public Health and Environmental Protection (RIVM) in the Netherlands. The RIVM is active in various fields of biomedical research, such as toxicology and pharmacology, and in the production and quality control of vaccines. Especially in the last-mentioned field, large numbers of animals are used. Detailed information is given on RIVM activities with respect to the development and validation of alternative methods in potency testing of bacterial vaccines.

Abbreviations. CAD = Center for Alternatives to Animal Testing; ELISA = enzyme-linked immunosorbent assay; RIVM = National Institute of Public Health and Environmental Protection; ToBI = toxin binding inhibition.

7.1 Introduction

Interest in alternatives to animal experiments has greatly increased in the last few years, also in the scientific world. Nevertheless, it must be concluded that actual research in this direction is generally given low priority by institute management and individual researchers, particularly when this research has a low scientific value. Efforts are being made to intensify activities in the field of Reduction, Replacement and Refinement, the so-called Three Rs, through the government, national centers for alternatives to animal testing, and numerous symposia and workshops. However, it appears that this approach reaches only the limited group of researchers who already recognize the need for research into alternatives and are active in this field. The majority of researchers, however, are too far removed from the stimulus of the appropriate bodies, and interest in alternatives seems destined to remain at its present level.

Alternatives to Animal Testing. New Ways in the Biomedical Sciences, Trends and Progress.
Reinhardt, C. A. (ed.). 1994. © VCH, Weinheim.

One possibility for making both institute management and individual researchers sensitive to the Three Rs and for initiating research in this field is the establishment of institute-linked centers for alternative methods. The importance of such centers, especially for the development of an institute policy and strategy in the field of animal experiments and alternatives to animal testing, must be emphasized. Only in this way can an atmosphere be created within an institute where working on the Three Rs is regarded as a matter of course.

An institute-linked center for alternatives has been operating within the National Institute of Public Health and Environmental Protection (RIVM) in Bilthoven, the Netherlands, for several years. The objectives, structure, and activities of this center will be elucidated in this paper. In the field of vaccine quality control, projects have been set up within the RIVM to reduce and refine the use of animals. This has already produced a number of concrete results, which will also be discussed.

7.2   Conditions for the development of alternatives

In general, a number of conditions have to be fulfilled before an alternative method can be developed. In a nutshell, these are: a competent researcher or team of researchers interested in the Three Rs and working in a well-equipped laboratory; an idea that can be implemented technically and scientifically; the financial means; and, finally, an institute management that attaches importance to this type of research. Factors that may impede the development of alternatives are shown schematically in Figure 7-1.

The development and use of alternative methods within an institution can be stimulated through a purposive government policy, social pressure, and the provision of funds. This brings to mind, for example, the EC legislation on animal testing, especially Article 23, which has already led to the setting up of ECVAM (European Centre for the Validation of Alternative Methods) in the laboratory of the Community's Joint Research Centre at Ispra, Italy. Other examples are the "national" centers for alternatives such as FRAME, SIAT, or ZEBET, organizations which coordinate and fund research on alternatives. All these activities contribute to a change of attitudes whereby the Three Rs receive the attention they deserve.

Although researchers and institute management are nowadays generally favorably disposed towards the goals of the Three Rs, many of them do not embark upon research because concrete impulses are lacking. Only in those cases in which the development of alternatives has a clear scientific and/or economic value will activities in this direction be developed. In the pharmaceutical industry, for example, animals are increasingly being replaced by in vitro techniques, such as organ preparations or cellular fractions, for the primary screening of drugs (de Jonge et al., 1991). For those fields that are scientifically and/or economically less interesting, however, the development and introduction of alternatives does not materialize because of the low priority given to them. An illustrative example can be found in the quality control of vaccines (Hendriksen, 1991). As far back as the 1960s, an in vitro model was described (Izbicky, 1968) for determining the amount of neutralizing antibodies against diphtheria in serum by titration. On the basis of validation studies, a good correlation was found to exist between the in vitro method and the accepted in vivo neutralization test (in guinea pigs). Nevertheless, the in vivo method was used in the potency testing of diphtheria vaccines until well into the eighties owing to the lack of any stimulus to limit the use of animals. It was not until 1985 that the in vitro test was modified and introduced into vaccine potency testing in the

Development of alternative

Causes of stagnation in alternatives research

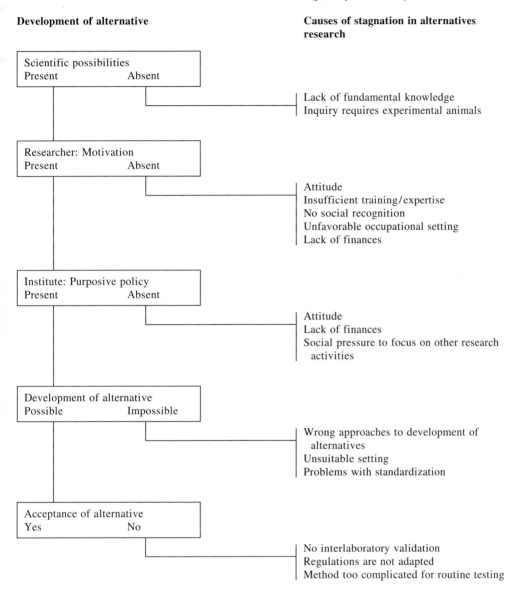

Figure 7-1. Causes of stagnation in alternatives research.

Netherlands (Kreeftenberg *et al.*, 1985). It is a sad fact that most countries still base their potency testing of diphtheria vaccines on the in vivo challenge test.

One possibility of breaking the passivity with regard to the Three Rs is the setting up of centers at the institute level, whose aim is to further the development, acceptance, and use of alternatives within the institution. This approach to the alternatives issue has a number of advantages:

– A change of attitude can be brought about from within the institute, which is usually very effective. In this context it is important that the institute's management defines a clear policy and strategy on replacement, reduction, and refinement.

– A direct appeal can be made to individual researchers. Researchers can be actively encouraged to develop and apply alternative methods and can be supported in their activities. In addition, researchers can be sent as representatives to expert committees of regulatory bodies such as the European Pharmacopoeia, the World Health Organization, or the Organization for Economic Cooperation and Development. This makes it possible to influence directly the regulations relating to testing in accordance with standard protocols.

– A central information point is created within the institute.

– Knowledge of the institute's structure enables a correct assessment of the feasibility of research into alternative methods.

Experience with such an institute-linked center has already been gained over the last few years at the RIVM.

7.3   The RIVM Center for Alternatives to Animal Testing (CAD)

The National Institute of Public Health and Environmental Protection (RIVM) in Bilthoven has about 1600 employees. It carries out research and advises the government on factors influencing public health and the environment. Within this context, the RIVM is active in the fields of microbiology, immunology, pharmacology, toxicology, and chemistry. In addition, the RIVM is responsible for the production and quality control of vaccines used in the National Vaccination Program in the Netherlands.

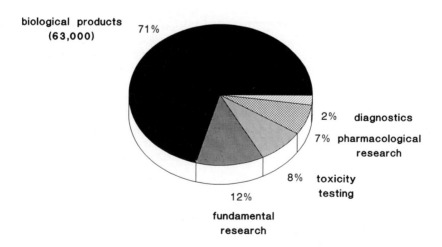

Total use of laboratory animals: 88,700

Figure 7-2. Use of laboratory animals at the National Institute of Public Health and Environmental Protection (RIVM) in 1990.

With 88 700 animals in 1990, the RIVM is one of the largest of the 90 animal-using institutions in the Netherlands (total number of animals used in the Netherlands in 1990: 951 000). Figure 7-2 gives a breakdown of animal use within the RIVM according to the purpose of the experiment. Most of the animals (63 000, about 71%) were required for the quality control of vaccines.

The RIVM's policy is to reduce the use of animals within the Institute even more than is already the case, and to this end the Directorate decided in 1991 to set up an institute-linked center for alternatives to animal testing (CAD). One condition was that this center should not have a narrow focus, but that as many RIVM departments as possible should be involved in the activities. A structure was chosen according to which the various departments of the Institute are represented in the center by a contact person. These contact persons are expected to be alert to the developments within their speciality and, in consultation with the center, to initiate projects and/or introduce methods which could lead to a reduction and refinement in animal experiments. The relevant activities take place within the participating departments. There are two staff members who coordinate the activities of the center, with a budget of $60 000 at their disposal. This budget is mainly intended for additional financing of projects and not for primary financing.

Furthermore, an Advisory Committee has been set up, consisting of six researchers of standing in the Institute, whose task it is to monitor and further the activities of the center, and also to help give direction to the Institute's policy. In practice, the Advisory Committee is proving to be extremely valuable, as its members, all of whom have a central and leading position within the Institute, exert a stimulating influence upon the other staff members.

In broad terms, the CAD concentrates on activities that can lead to a reduction and/or refinement of laboratory animal use:

– It initiates research on the development or validation of alternative methods, in collaboration with the researcher(s) involved.
– It provides additional funds for the development, validation, and application of alternative methods. The projects which were financially supported in 1991 are listed in Table 7-1.
– It encourages the use of existing alternative methods, for example, through measures which create suitable conditions, such as the establishment of a central facility for the production of monoclonal antibodies, which resulted in the almost complete replacement of animal use for this purpose by in vitro methods.
– It stimulates interest in the goals of the Three Rs through incentives such as the creation and awarding of an Institute-linked prize.

Table 7-1. Projects on alternatives financially supported by the RIVM Center for Alternatives in 1991.

–   Evaluation of alternatives to complete Freunds adjuvant (FCA)

–   Use of liver slices to study the metabolism of xenobiotics

–   Improvement of in vitro monoclonal production

–   ELISA techniques as an alternative to in vivo potency test for rabies vaccine

–   Cytokine release test as an in vitro alternative to in vivo pyrogenicity test

–   Modification of procedures for laboratory animal anesthesia and analgesia

– It publicizes the concept of *alternatives to animal tests* among a large group of researchers through activities such as the organization of symposia and conferences, and the publication of a periodical newsletter.
– It advises staff members on the welfare of experimental animals and on alternatives to animal tests.

Although the center has been in existence for only a few years, it may nevertheless be concluded that it fills a need, and numerous activities have been started in the field of the Three Rs. The following outline of the activities involving vaccine control illustrates the research into alternatives carried out within the RIVM. The quality control of vaccines, required by law, requires especially large numbers of animals. The tests are usually performed in accordance with a standard protocol based on the guidelines of the European Pharmacopoeia and WHO.

7.4   Alternatives in the quality control of vaccines

A breakdown of the use of animals within the RIVM for the quality control of vaccines by type of test is given in Table 7-2. It can be seen that the majority of the animals are required for potency testing. Since the potency testing of live vaccines is based on in vitro models, the entire use is for the potency testing of inactivated vaccines. At the RIVM, they are the diphtheria, tetanus, pertussis, poliomyelitis, and rabies vaccines.

In general, potency tests consist of quantitative bioassays, which measure the protective immunizing capacity of vaccine batches by means of a challenge procedure with the virulent organism.

Table 7-2. Number of animals required and distress rating for the various tests used in the quality control of diphtheria, tetanus, and pertussis vaccines in the Netherlands in 1985.

Animal test	Approx. no. of animals	Distress rating[a]
Potency[b]	46 213	severe
Specific toxicity	1 200	slight to severe
Abnormal toxicity	250	slight

[a] See van Zutphen, this volume, for an explanation of distress ratings.
[b] Data on the potency test are based on the lethal challenge procedure.

7.4.1   Potency test in vaccine quality control: opportunities for replacement, reduction, and refinement

To illustrate the possibilities of the Three Rs in biomedical research, the potency testing of the inactivated human vaccines forms an excellent starting point. In the traditional potency test, which is still used on a large scale, two stages can be distinguished. In the first stage, groups of animals are immunized with dilutions of the vaccine being tested or of a standard preparation. After a given immunization period, the second stage, the so-called challenge, begins, in which animals are injected with the virulent organism or toxin. On the basis of mortality in the various animal groups, the efficacy of the vaccine under test can then be expressed in units of the standard preparation using a statistical computer program. A project was started in the mid-eighties at the RIVM with the ultimate goal of reducing and refining the use of animals in the potency testing of bacterial vaccines, starting with diphtheria and tetanus toxoid. Several approaches were studied. These possibilities are discussed briefly.

Until a few years ago, the accepted number of animals used per vaccine dilution in potency testing was 16 or more. This number was based on the requirements of the European Pharmacopoeia and the WHO that the number of animals should be sufficient to ensure a 95 % confidence interval within the range 50–200 % of the estimated potency. We were able to show that the 50–200 % requirement could still be met with only half the number of animals, i. e. 10 animals per vaccine dilution (Hendriksen *et al.*, 1987). The WHO (WHO, 1990) guidelines have in the meantime been adapted to the effect that the minimum number of animals may be reduced when consistency of production and testing has been established.

The current potency tests are based on a quantitative approach, in which three dilutions of a test preparation are compared with three dilutions of a reference preparation. This so-called *3 + 3* assay is a statistically valid test, giving reliable and accurate results, also when using a reduced number of animals for each vaccine dose. However, it might be and has been questioned whether accurate results are required, since the estimates of potency should exceed a specified number of international units. Present-day toxoid vaccines are potent and defined products, and consistency of production has been established at most production centers. Therefore, a simplified potency test for the routine control of diphtheria and tetanus toxoid batches was evaluated. We evaluated a simplified test based on a *1 + 1* assay, in which one group of animals (e. g. 12 animals) is immunized with one dose of the vaccine being tested and one group of animals with one dose of the reference preparation. Evaluation showed that this test, at least in our hands, was a valid approach to show that the vaccine batch exceeded the minimum requirements (Akkermans *et al.*, 1993; Marsman *et al.*, 1993).

Alternatives to the lethal challenge procedure in vaccine potency testing have been described. The amount of toxin-neutralizing antibodies induced after immunization is no longer determined by means of a lethal challenge but by the bleeding of the animals under anesthesia followed by serum titration in in vitro assay systems. A cell culture test has been developed at our institute for the diphtheria potency assay and a modified ELISA assay, the toxin binding inhibition (ToBI) test, for the tetanus potency assay.

Apart from diphtheria and tetanus potency testing, Three Rs research is also under study at the RIVM for the potency assay on rabies vaccines and pertussis vaccines (Table 7-3).

In summary, it can be stated that for the potency testing of vaccines there are various possibilities for considerably refining and/or reducing the use of animals.

Table 7-3. Three Rs research in vaccine quality control (potency testing) at the RIVM.

Vaccine	Alternative model
Rabies	In vitro antigenicity test (ELISA)
Pertussis	Serology (ELISA)
Diphtheria	Reduction in numbers of animals Serology (VERO cells) Single dilution assay Use of F1-hybrid animals
Tetanus	Serology (ToBI) Reduction in numbers of animals

7.5   Conclusion

By adopting an innovative as well as an evaluative approach with regard to the Three Rs, we have succeeded in reducing substantially the numbers of animals used at our institute for the quality control of bacterial vaccines. To outline the reductions achieved: The routine application at our institute of in vitro assay systems as an alternative to the lethal challenge procedure reduced both the number of animals (about 3000 a year) and the degree of distress caused to animals. Statistical re-assessment of the numbers of animals required for potency testing of batches of toxoid vaccines resulted in an annual reduction of about 5000 animals. In addition, the in vitro ToBI test has been replaced by the in vivo assay for the estimation of tetanus and diphtheria antitoxin in human sera, resulting in a reduction of about 8000 mice and 300 guinea-pigs a year.

References

Akkermans A. A., Hendriksen C. F. M., Marsman F. R., de Jong W. H. and v. d. Donk H. J. M. (1993) *Evaluation of a Single Dilution Potency Assay Based upon Serology of Vaccines Containing Diphtheria Toxoid: Analysis for Consistency in Production and Testing at the Laboratory for the Control of Biological Products of the R. I. V. M.* (RIVM Report no. 172203001). RIVM, Bilthoven, the Netherlands.

Hendriksen C. F. M. (1991) The use of animals in the production and quality control of biologicals: current practice and possible alternatives. In *Animals in Biomedical Research, Replacement, Reduction and Refinement: Present Possibilities and Future Prospects.* Edited by C.F.M. Hendriksen and H. B. W. M. Koëter. pp. 49–68. Elsevier Science Publishers B. V., Amsterdam.

Hendriksen C. F. M., van der Gun J. W., Marsman F. R. and Kreeftenberg J. G. (1987) The effects of reductions in the numbers of animals used for the potency assay of the diphtheria and tetanus components of adsorbed vaccines by the methods of the European Pharmacopoeia. *Journal of Biological Standardization* **15**, 353–362.

Izbicky A. (1968) Titration von Diphtherie-Toxin und Antitoxin auf Grund des zytopathischen Effektes in der BSC-1 Zellkultur. *Zeitschrift für Immunitätsforschung* **136**, 415–420.

Jonge R. de, Reinders J. H. and Pereboom W. J. (1991) The role of animal experiments and alternatives in industrial pharmacological research. In *Animals in Biomedical Research, Replacement, Reduction and Refinement: Present Possibilities and Future Prospects.* Edited by C.F.M. Hendriksen and H. B. W. M. Koëter. pp. 101–111. Elsevier Science Publishers B. V., Amsterdam.

Kreeftenberg J. G., van der Gun J. W., Marsman F. R., Sekhuis V. M., Bhandari S. K. and Maheswari S. C. (1985) An investigation of a mouse model to estimate the potency of the diphtheria component in combined vaccines. *Journal of Biological Standardization* **13**, 229–234.

Marsman F. R., Akkermans A. A., Hendriksen C. F. M. and de Jong W. H. (1993) *Evaluation of a Single Dilution Potency Assay Based upon Serology of Vaccines Containing Diphtheria Toxoid: Statistical Analysis* (RIVM Report no. 172203002). RIVM, Bilthoven, the Netherlands.

World Health Organization (1990) *Requirements for Diphtheria, Tetanus, Pertussis and Combined Vaccines* (revised 1989) (WHO Technical Report Series). WHO, Geneva.

8 ZEBET: Three Years of the National German Center for Documentation and Evaluation of Alternatives to Animal Experiments at the Federal Health Office (BGA) in Berlin

Horst Spielmann, Barbara Grune-Wolff, and Manfred Liebsch

Summary

In 1989, the Center for Documentation and Evaluation of Alternative Methods to Animal Experiments (ZEBET) was established at the Institute of Veterinary Medicine of the Federal Health Office (BGA) in Berlin. ZEBET 1 is responsible for documentation and information on alternatives to animal experiments, including an alternatives databank. ZEBET 2 serves as national center for planning, funding, and coordinating validation programs for alternative test methods, such as new methods of determining acute toxicity (LD_{50}), eye irritation (Draize test), and fish toxicity. ZEBET 3 has laboratory facilities both for participation in validation studies and for visiting scientists, who can participate in developing new experimental approaches to replace, reduce, and refine the current use of experimental animals.

Abbreviations. BGA = Federal Health Office; BMFT = Department of Research and Technology; BMG = Department of Health; BML = Department of Agriculture; ZEBET = Center for Documentation and Evaluation of Alternative Methods to Animal Experiments.

8.1 Administrative organization of ZEBET

In the process of harmonizing the German Animal Protection Law (Tierschutzgesetz) with European legislation (Council Directive 86/609/EEC), the Center for Documentation and Evaluation of Alternative Methods to Animal Experiments (Zentralstelle zur Erfassung und Bewertung von Ersatz- und Ergänzungsmethoden zum Tierversuch, ZEBET) was established in 1989 at the Institute of Veterinary Medicine of the Federal Health Office (BGA = Bundesgesundheitsamt) in Berlin. ZEBET is responsible for the documentation of alternative methods and also for validation and acceptance of the new methods at the national and the international level, e. g. by the EC or OECD. At the international level, ZEBET cooperates with institutions with a similar scientific scope and ethical mission, such as CAAT (Baltimore, U.S.A.), FRAME (Nottingham, England), RIVM (Bilthoven, Netherlands), SIAT (Switzerland), and the new European Centre for the Validation of Alternative Methods, ECVAM (Ispra, Italy).

According to ZEBET's major activities in the fields of documentation/information, validation, and research, three units were formed: ZEBET 1, 2, and 3 (Figure 8-1).

Alternatives to Animal Testing. New Ways in the Biomedical Sciences, Trends and Progress.
Reinhardt, C. A. (ed.). 1994. © VCH, Weinheim.

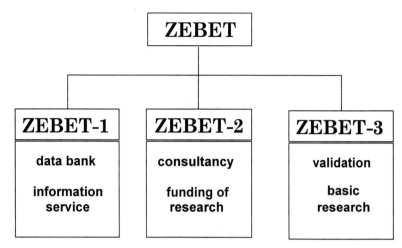

Figure 8-1. Organizational structure of ZEBET (National German Center for Documentation and Evaluation of Alternatives to Animal Experiments).

ZEBET 1 is responsible for documentation and information on alternatives to animal experiments. This includes establishing an alternatives databank. In addition, ZEBET serves as national and international information center on alternatives to animal experiments.

ZEBET 2 is the national administrative and scientific center for planning, funding, and coordinating validation programs that are aimed at reducing and replacing animal tests in regulatory toxicology and safety testing, such as new methods for determining acute toxicity (LD_{50}), eye irritation (Draize test), and fish toxicity. In close cooperation with the EC, ZEBET is engaged in managing and conducting validation studies at the international level. ZEBET has a small budget for funding research at the national level to develop alternative methods in collaboration with the German Ministry of Research and Technology (BMFT).

ZEBET 3 has laboratory facilities that not only enable ZEBET to participate in validation studies but also allow visiting scientists to develop new experimental approaches to replace, reduce, and refine the use of experimental animals in all areas of experimental biomedicine.

Some of the difficulties ZEBET has had to overcome at the administrative level result from the fact that ZEBET reports to three different departments (ministries) of the federal government in Bonn, as shown in Figure 8-2. As part of the Federal Health Office (BGA), the federal agency reporting to the Ministry of Health (BMG = Bundesministerium für Gesundheit), ZEBET is on the budgets of BMG and BGA, both of which have to ensure consumer protection.

In the federal government of Germany, the minister of agriculture (BML = Bundesministerium für Landwirtschaft) is responsible for all aspects of animal protection, including alternatives to the use of experimental animals. During the past three years ZEBET has, therefore, closely cooperated with the BML. Moreover, in the federal government of Germany the minister of research and technology (BMFT = Bundesministerium für Forschung und Technologie) is responsible for all aspects of research funding, including the development of alternatives to animal experiments. In establishing validation projects in Germany to evaluate the

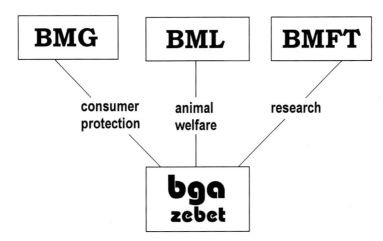

Figure 8-2. ZEBET's cooperation with federal ministries. BMG = Department of Health (Bundesministerium für Gesundheit); BML = Department of Agriculture (Bundesministerium für Landwirtschaft); BMFT = Department of Research and Technology (Bundesministerium für Forschung und Technologie); BGA = Federal Health Office (Bundesgesundheitsamt).

reproducibility of alternative methods ZEBET cooperates closely with the BMFT. It is obvious that this organizational structure, according to which ZEBET collaborates with and reports to both the BML and the BMFT and at the same time has to try to get funding from the BMG via the budget of the BGA, should be improved.

ZEBET's tenured staff increased from two in 1989, when it was established, to ten in 1991. However, since this staff is assigned only to ZEBET 1 and ZEBET 2, the staff of ZEBET 3, ranging from six to nine, has so far been funded with limited contracts from grants provided by either the BMFT or the EC. The improvement of the situation of the staff of ZEBET 3 has a high priority among the three federal ministries, BMG, BMFT and BML, as its experimental work, such as the development of new in vitro methods in toxicology and participation in national and international validation studies, is well appreciated.

8.2   The ZEBET alternatives databank

The ZEBET databank serves as an information service for scientists, government agencies, organizations, and the public, providing information on the current status of alternative methods to animal experiments. Therefore, establishing ZEBET represents a national attempt to actively promote the use of alternative methods instead of laboratory animals in biomedicine in Germany.

For this purpose, scientists at ZEBET not only document literature on alternative methods in the ZEBET databank, but also evaluate to what extent a particular method has been developed so as to serve the purpose of reducing, replacing, or refining (the Three Rs) a specific experimental procedure that requires the use of animals. The documentation of alternative methods in the ZEBET databank is, therefore, a two-stage process (Spielmann *et al.*, 1992).

In the first stage, literature is collected from original scientific publications, from searches in publicly accessible databanks like MEDLINE, and also directly from scientists who are using methods that have not been published in detail. The range of the search for alternative methods covers a broad spectrum of the biomedical sciences, including pharmacology and drug development, toxicology, cancer research and experimental medicine, microbiology, parasitology, physiology, immunology, endocrinology and neurology.

In the second stage, scientists at ZEBET evaluate whether an alternative method holds promise for the solution of scientific problems that could so far only be approached by using experimental animals, or to what extent new or modified procedures can serve to reduce the suffering of laboratory animals. Moreover, they attempt to evaluate what kind of additional experimental evidence has to be provided to achieve the acceptance of a new method as an alternative for an established experimental animal model both at the national and at the international level. The result of the evaluation and a short description of the method are presented in a summary.

For the reasons outlined above, the information in the ZEBET databank includes the following:

– a description of a specific alternative method (aim, Three R-principle, endpoints);
– an evaluation of the method according to the Three R-principles of Russell and Burch (1959): *replace, reduce, refine*;
– a description of the animal experiment that can be replaced, reduced, or refined;
– the names of scientists who are experienced in the field of the specific alternative method;
– references to literature on the specific alternative method and on the animal experiment to be replaced, reduced, or refined.

This information is stored in the ZEBET databank for each method and will constantly be updated to be available through the ZEBET information service. In answering inquiries, the ZEBET information service consults not only the ZEBET databank but also other publicly accessible databanks such as MEDLINE, EMBASE, and INVITTOX. An overview of the current in vitro toxicology databanks is given in Table 8-1. It is important to note that the ZEBET databank as well as most of the other new in vitro toxicology databanks provides information on ongoing validation studies.

According to current planning, the ZEBET databank and information service will serve not only Germany but also Austria and Switzerland. Most of the information in the ZEBET databank is available only in German, however, both the summary and the list of references are given in English.

During the past three years, ZEBET'S information service has provided predominantly administrative information to animal protection officers, government agencies, scientific institutions, and industry.

Table 8-1. Current in vitro toxicology databanks.

Project name and sponsor	Purpose of databank (hardware)	Area of application	Contact person	Reference
Gelbe Liste (Yellow List) German Acad. f. Anim. Protect. (est. 1987)	Collection of in vitro methods (PC)	Research & testing, pharm., tox., **validation**	**B. Rusche** Akademie für Tierschutz, Munich, Germany	Rusche, 1989
INVITTOX ERGATT/CEC & FRAME (est. 1988)	Collection of in vitro methods (PC)	Research & testing, pharm., tox., **validation**	**K. Ungar** c/o FRAME, Nottingham England	Warren *et al.*, 1989
Register of Cytotoxicity private & acad. Science (est. 1988)	300 chemicals mammalian cyto-toxicity IC_{50} data & acute LD_{50} (book)	Research & testing, pharm., tox.	**W. Halle** Inst. Molec. Drug Research Berlin, Germany	Halle and Göres, 1988
ALTDBASE Japan. Res. Group Alt. to Anim. Testing (est. 1989)	In vitro tests experimental data (PC)	Research & testing, pharm., tox.	**Y. Yamada** Natl. Inst. Radiol. Sci. Japan	Yamada, 1990
ZEBET German Fed. Health Office BGA (est. 1989)	In vitro tests methods and experimental data (PC)	Research & testing, pharm., tox. bact, immun. **validation**	**H. Spielmann** ZEBET, BGA, Berlin, Germany	Spielmann, 1989; Spielmann *et al.*, 1992
IVT/DCI Technical Database Services (est. 1990)	In vitro tox. testing database ongoing valida-tion projects (PC)	Research & testing, pharm., tox., **validation**	**M. Green** Technical Data-base Services New York	IVT, 1992
GALILEO DATA BANK CEC/Univ. Pisa (est. 1990)	In vitro tox., genotoxicity, carcinogenicity (PC)	Research & testing, pharm., tox.,	**N. Loprieno** Biological Research Planning, (BRP) Pisa, Italy	Loprieno *et al.*, 1991
Open access databanks operating worldwide				
MEDLINE U.S. Natl. Lib. Med.	Biomedical literature databank (on-line)	Research & experimental **unspecific**	Worldwide access	Local inform. centers
RTECS TOXNET. TOXLINE U.S. Natl. Lib. Med.	Toxicology literature databank (on-line)	Research & experimental **unspecific**	Worldwide access	Local inform. centers
TOPCAT Health Sci. Inc. U.S.A.	Predict. tox endpoints from chem. struct. (PC)	Testing & research **unspecific**	Commercial product	Health Sci. Inc. Bethesda, U.S.A.

8.3   ZEBET's funding of research on alternatives

One of the tasks of ZEBET is to stimulate research aimed at developing and validating methods that reduce both the suffering and use of experimental animals. This is achieved, on the one hand, through research projects carried out in the ZEBET 3 laboratory, which so far has been financed strictly by external funds from either the German BMFT or the EC (DG XI and XII). On the other hand, ZEBET has been funding research on alternatives at the national level since 1990 with the stipulation that the research be carried out outside the BGA. The annual amount for this in ZEBET's budget has increased from DM 400000 in 1990 to DM 600000 in 1992.

A comparison with the other two governmental sources of funding of research in this field is given in Table 8-2. It shows that this item in the annual budget of the BMFT is about

Table 8-2. Governmental sources of funding of research on alternatives to animal experiments in Germany.

Source	Amount per year
BMFT (Department of Research and Technology) 1990–1992	DM 5000000
Baden-Württemberg 1989–1991	DM 750000
ZEBET/BGA 1990–1992	DM 400000–600000

ten times higher than that of ZEBET and of Baden-Württemberg, the only German state supporting research in this field. It provides an amount similar to ZEBET's annual funding budget. Cooperation and an exchange of information takes place between ZEBET and the funding committees of the BMFT and of Baden-Württemberg. Furthermore, it was decided at ZEBET to support a larger group of small but promising projects rather than a few large projects. Thus many of the small projects supported by ZEBET have a chance to progress and obtain funding by more potent sponsors both at the national level, e. g. BMFT, and at the international level, e. g. EC.

The following criteria are used to evaluate applications of grant proposals submitted to ZEBET for funding:

– The effects on animal welfare in terms of the amount of suffering and number of animals used in the animal experiment to be replaced, reduced, or refined;
– The scientific merit of the experimental approach;
– The state of validation according to the criteria of the Amden report (Balls *et al.*, 1990), including a decision on the application as a screening or adjunct test;
– The coordination of funding with other agencies both at the national and the international level.

After the first announcement of the new ZEBET funding program in 1990, 27 applications were submitted, and another 29 proposals followed the second advertisement in 1992. In 1990 and also in 1992, funds could be provided for grant applications either for scientific equipment only (5 of the projects in 1990; 5 in 1992) or for laboratory staff (7 of the projects in 1990; 6 in 1992).

A short summary shows that projects funded by ZEBET cover a broad spectrum of the biomedical sciences:

Validation of new in vitro tests in toxicology
– fish cell cytotoxicity assay to replace a fish test that is used in Germany routinely for monitoring waste water;
– in vitro biocompatibility testing of biomaterials.

Development of new bioassays
– in vitro determination of calcitonin;
– immunological batch control of the potency of *Erysipelothrix rhusiopathiae* vaccine.

Development of new endpoints for in vitro cytotoxicity
– heat-shock proteins as indicator of toxic stress;
– videomicroscopy of intracellular changes of proteins due to toxic stress.

In vitro screening in drug development
– interaction between receptors and cardiac drugs in human heart tissue obtained from cardiac surgery;
– testing of cardiac drugs on spontaneously beating heart muscle cells derived from mouse embryonic stem cells.

Structure-activity relationships (SAR)
– SAR of valproic acid enantiomeres as model drugs to predict embryotoxic potential of drugs.

Use of genetically engineered permanent cell lines to replace animal testing
– stable expression of human P450 cytochromes in V79 cells for predicting human biotransformation in vitro;
– stable (over)-expression of human β-adrenergic receptors in CHO cells for receptor binding studies.

Some of the studies funded by ZEBET have gained international recognition through being awarded prestigious alternatives research prizes, for example, the projects on embryonic stem cells and on genetically engineered permanent cells lines. Moreover, several of the projects were successful in obtaining broader funding by the BMFT or EC.

8.4   ZEBET's validation activities

At present ZEBET 3 is experimentally involved in four national and international validation projects. One of these is a national validation study on alternatives to the Draize rabbit's eye test, two are international studies on the same subject, and the fourth is an international validation trial on different in vitro phototoxicity assays.

Between 1988 and 1992, a national validation study on two alternatives to the Draize eye test was conducted in 14 laboratories in Germany. It was funded by the BMFT and coordinated by ZEBET. Results of the stages of intra- and interlaboratory assessment and interlaboratory assessment, the first two stages of this validation trial, have already been published (Kalweit *et al.*, 1990; Spielmann *et al.*, 1991).

During database development, the last stage of validation according to the Amden workshop (Balls *et al.*, 1990), 136 chemicals from the German chemical industry were classified in a blind trial with the 3T3 cell neutral red/kenacid blue cytotoxicity assay and the HET-CAM test using embryonated chicken eggs (Kalweit *et al.*, 1990). In vivo Draize eye testing data were provided by industry, and the test chemicals were selected to represent a wide spectrum of chemical structures and toxicological properties. Not unexpectedly, it was impossible to correlate cytotoxicity data with the EC classification of in vivo eye irritation data. However, the majority of severely irritating chemicals (labelling R-41) could be identified correctly in the HET-CAM assay, whereas test conditions did not allow identification of irritating chemicals (R-36). The HET-CAM test, therefore, fulfills the criteria of a *well-validated alternative method* according to OECD guideline 405 (OECD, 1987) and should be incorporated into eye irritation testing at the earliest stage possible to effectively reduce the suffering of rabbits in the Draize eye test (Spielmann *et al.*, 1993).

The second validation study in which ZEBET has participated was funded by the DG XI of the EC. Towards replacing the Draize rabbit's eye test, isolated bovine cornea from the slaughter house were tested in a blind validation trial in 12 laboratories in 5 European countries with 52 selected test chemicals. Results will be presented in 1993.

It is difficult to decide from the results of the many validation studies that have been carried out worldwide which of the systems will be accepted as an alternative to the Draize eye test at the international level. The DG XI of the EC has, therefore, decided to fund and coordinate an international validation study of the most promising alternatives to this test. This validation study will cover nine alternatives that are established in laboratories of the European chemical industry. Each test will be performed in at least four different laboratories in Europe and the U.S.A., and 60 coded chemicals will be tested blind. Owing to its experience in the coordination of validation studies, ZEBET is involved in the planning and management of this project. It is scheduled to begin early in 1993, and results are expected within 18 months.

Photoirritancy is an area in which in vitro models using human or animal tissue seem to be more promising than any of the animal models developed so far. To test the evidence suggested by preliminary data, the DG XI of the EC and the European Cosmetics Manufacturers Association (COLIPA) started a joint validation project of in vitro photoirritation tests in 1992. ZEBET is managing and participating in this validation trial with seven other laboratories from four European countries. The study is focused on in vitro methods that are established in laboratories of the European cosmetics industry as well as on test systems that are commercially available. The photoirritancy study is scheduled for the years 1992–1994.

8.5   ZEBET's activities in Germany after unification in 1990

Animal rights was not an important ethical or scientific issue in the former East Germany (GDR), and a funding program for research aimed at developing alternatives to the use of experimental animals did not exist. Immediately after the fall of the Berlin wall at the end of 1989, scientists from the former GDR tried to establish contact with ZEBET, as up to that time the open exchange of scientific information had been illegal. Already before the official uni-fication of Germany in October, 1990, ZEBET helped scientists from the GDR obtain infor-mation on literature, on the funding of research on tissue culture techniques, and on the use of alternatives. In 1990–1991, ZEBET was able to start funding research in several laboratories in the former GDR, and subsequently in 1991–1992 ZEBET was successful in initiating col-laborative research projects between scientists in the former GDR and scientists from univer-sities and/or industry in the former West Germany, funded by the BMFT.

To promote the concepts of the Three Rs according to Russell and Burch (1959) in the former GDR in the areas of research, teaching, and regulatory safety testing, ZEBET has held seminars on the use and development of alternatives in collaboration with animal protection officers and universities in the five "new German states," including East Berlin.

It should not be overlooked that in some fields of biomedical research, methods had been developed by scientists in the former GDR independently from "Western" science that were scientifically more advanced, as, for example, the in vitro culture and differentiation of mammalian embryonic stem cells by Anna Wobus in Gatersleben and the production of poly-clonal avian anibodies by Rüdiger Schade in East Berlin. Finally, Willi Halle from East Berlin deserves mention, as it was he who founded the German Society for Cell and Tissue Culture (GZG) 20 years ago, much earlier than the establishment of a similar society in West Germany. Because Dr. Halle did not support the political system of the GDR, he could not pursue his studies on cyctotoxicity the way he had started them more than 20 years ago. Although he was well over 60 when the wall came down, he was pleased that his basic ideas had in the meantime been accepted by most of his Western colleagues. It was, therefore, a spe-cial privilege for scientists at ZEBET to be able to fund his research already in 1990 and to help him publish some of his basic papers in internationally recognized journals (Halle *et al.*, 1991; Halle and Spielmann, 1992).

8.6   ZEBET's outlook

During its first years, ZEBET had to define and find its position inside the Federal Health Institute (BGA) at the national level and, in particular, at the international level inside and beyond the EC. The struggle to get established and funded in a regulatory agency was not easy. However, when ZEBET got its own budget for the fiscal year 1993, an important step towards independence was reached.

At the European and at the international level ZEBET has been privileged, as it is one of the few government institutions in the in vitro sciences. The cooperation with new institu-tions, such as ECVAM, will help ZEBET to promote the development, validation, and accep-tance of new in vitro methods. Initiated by the criticism of the use of laboratory animals in developing cosmetics, a successful cooperation has been established in the field of photoirri-tancy testing with the European cosmetics industry (COLIPA) and ECVAM. In a similar manner, ZEBET and ECVAM are engaged in the management of a worldwide validation study on alternatives to the Draize rabbit's eye test as well as in cooperating with the U.S. Inter Regulatory Agency Group (IRAG) to establish criteria for the evaluation of in vitro eye irritation tests.

Personal contacts have been vital in establishing cooperation among scientists in indus-try, academia, and regulatory agencies to promote the concept of alternatives to animal test-ing. However, these activities would have been impossible without the stimulating support of individual citizens, who have felt, for example, that the use of animals in safety testing for consumer protection is outdated in an age when human fertilization and embryo culture can be successfully performed in vitro. And, although we are indeed grateful for this support, we still ask for more support and patience, as the way ahead is still steep and rough.

Acknowledgements. Establishing ZEBET as a government agency inside the national German Federal Health Office (BGA) as well as its expansion and permanent funding would not have been possible without the permanent support of the political parties of our parliament and of the organizations and individuals in our country who have identified alternatives to animal experiments as an important political, ethical and scientific challenge of our decade.

References

Balls M., Blaauboer B., Brusik D., Frazier J., Lamp D., Pemberton M., Reinhardt C., Robertfroid M., Rosenkranz H., Schmid B., Spielmann H., Stammati A. L. and Walum E. (1990) Report and recommendations of the CAAT/ERGATT workshop on the validation of toxicity test procedures. *ATLA* **18,** 313–337.

Halle W., Baeger I., Ekwall B. and Spielmann H. (1991) Correlation between in vitro cytotoxicity and octanol/water partition coefficient of 29 substances from the MEIC programme. *ATLA* **19,** 338–343.

Halle W. and Göres E. (1988) Register der Zytotoxizität (IC_{50}) in der Zellkultur und Möglichkeiten zur Abschätzung der akuten Toxizität (LD_{50}). *Beiträge zur Wirkstofforschung* **32,** 1–108.

Halle W. and Spielmann H. (1992) Two procedures for the prediction of acute toxicity (LD50) from cytotoxicity data. *ATLA* **20,** 40–49.

IVT (1992) *In Vitro* Toxicity Data Collection. *The Alternatives Report* **4,** 4.

Kalweit S., Besoke K., Gerner I. and Spielmann H. (1990) A national validation project of alternative methods to the Draize rabbit eye test. *Toxicology in Vitro* **4,** 702–706.

Loprieno N., Boncristiani G., Loprieno G. and Tesoro M. (1991) Data selection and treatment of chemicals tested for genotoxicity and carcinogenicity. *Environmental Health Perspectives* **96,** 121–126.

Organisation for Economic Cooperation and Development (1987) *OECD Guidelines for Testing of Chemicals. Test Guideline 405, Acute Eye Irritation/Corrosion.* OECD Publications Office, Paris.

Rusche B. (1989) Die Datenbank des Deutschen Tierschutzbundes e. V. *BGA Schriften* **2,** 68–72.

Russell W. M. S. and Burch R. L. (1959) *Principles of Humane Experimental Technique.* Methuen, London.

Spielmann H. (1989) Die Zentrale Erfassungs- und Bewertungsstelle für Ersatz- und Ergänzungsmethoden zum Tierversuch: Zielsetzung – Organisation – Planung. *Bundesgesundheitsblatt* **32,** 360–363.

Spielmann H., Gerner I., Kalweit S., Moog R., Wirnsberger T., Krauser K., Kreiling R., Kreuzer H., Lüpke N. P., Miltenburger H. G., Müller N., Mürmann P., Pape W., Siegemund B., Spengler J., Steiling W. and Wiebel F. (1991) Interlaboratory assessment of alternatives to the Draize eye irritation test in Germany. *Toxicology in Vitro* **5,** 539–542.

Spielmann H., Grune-Wolff B., Ewe S., Skolik S., Liebsch M., Traue D. and Heuer J. (1992) ZEBET's data bank and information service on alternatives to the use of experimental animals in Germany. *ATLA* **20,** 362–367.

Spielmann H., Kalweit S., Liebsch M., Wirnsberger T., Gerner I., Bertram-Neis E., Krauser K., Kreiling R., Miltenburger H., Pape W. and Steiling W. (1993) Validation study of alternatives to the Draize eye irritation test in Germany: cytotoxicity testing and HET-CAM assay with 136 industrial chemicals. *Toxicology in Vitro* **7,** 505–510.

Warren M., Atkinson K. and Steer S. (1989) Introducing INVITTOX: The ERGATT/FRAME *In Vitro* Toxicology Data Bank. *ATLA* **16,** 332–343.

Yamada T. (1990) Introducing ALTDBASE: Data base on the references of alternatives of animal testing. *Alternatives to Animal Testing and Experimentation* **1,** 42.

9 Reviewed Literature Databank for Alternatives to Animal Experiments – "Gelbe Liste"

Brigitte Rusche and Ursula G. Sauer

Summary

With the goal of countering prevailing neglect in the field of research on alternatives to animal experiments and of promoting the development of alternatives by pursuing projects of its own, the German Animal Welfare Association has installed a reviewed-literature PC-based databank for alternatives to animal experiments at the Academy for the Protection of Animals (Akademie für Tierschutz). The records in the databank are based on scientific papers; presently 10000 entries are stored according to a given scheme. With the help of defined key words, each publication is characterized according to certain aspects, so that it can be called up together with other similar publications in the process of a literature search. Information from the databank is available to anyone: scientists, public authorities, and animal rightists. Literature searches are performed on any given theme without a fee, and requests are processed without delay. University libraries and other institutions may obtain the entire databank along with regular updates.

9.1 Introduction

Not only the research on alternatives to animal experiments in general, but also the development of specific alternatives and the establishment of the use of existing in vitro methods is proceeding rather slowly. Therefore the German Animal Welfare Association (Deutscher Tierschutzbund e. V.) has recognized the necessity of calling attention to this prevailing neglect and of promoting the development of alternatives by pursuing projects of its own. As a contribution toward this goal, in 1986 the German Animal Welfare Association began working on a databank at the Academy for the Protection of Animals.

9.2 Description of the databank

The entries into the databank provide information about scientific publications. With permission of the author, unpublished studies are also included, thus giving a complete overview of the current state of research on alternative methods. A single document record in the databank is subdivided into different fields. Basic data are provided concerning the authors, the year of

Alternatives to Animal Testing. New Ways in the Biomedical Sciences, Trends and Progress.
Reinhardt, C. A. (ed.). 1994. © VCH, Weinheim.

publication, the reference, and the title. Additional fields are designed to characterize the subject and the method of a study. The characterization is done with regard to the aim of the databank, that is to reveal possibilities for the replacement of animal experiments by alternative methods. Each record is structured according to the scheme depicted in Figure 9-1.

The example shown in Figure 9-2 helps to illustrate such an entry. A publication by Buzaleh and co-authors dating from 1988 is documented. The study was published in the journal *ATLA* and has the stated title. This basic information is followed by a summary that describes the aim of the study.

Since it is not the purpose of the database to replace a scientist's study of the literature, information is not provided on scientific details. Instead, our summary points out in which manner a study can make a contribution to the replacement of animal experiments. Thus the example suggests that animal experiments involving the determination and examination of pharmaceutical substances whose side effects show that they interfere with metabolic processes and lead to an unwanted accumulation of porphyrines in various organs might be replaced by the in vitro method described. The results mentioned in the study are encouraging and make further evaluations advisable.

By means of *defined key words*, based on the thesaurus, each publication is indexed in several ways so that it may be selected together with other similar publications in the process of a literature search. The thesaurus, comprising the entirety of key words, is subdivided into five different descriptor groups to characterize the:

Basic Information
Author
Co-authors
Year of publication
Source
Title

Reviewed Information on the Study
Summary
Key words
Endpoint of the method
Special characterization

Additional Information
Address of the author
Call number

Internal Information
Entry date
Critical evaluation

Figure 9-1. The fields of a document record in the databank.

Buzaleh, A.M.; Afonso, S.G.; Polo, C.F.; Navone, N.M.; Bianchi, A.; Schoua, E.; Del C. Batlle, A.M.; Vázquez, E.S.
1988
ATLA 16/2: 137–144
Induction of porphyrin biosynthesis in the non-animal experimental model of tissue explant cultures: Prevention and reversal by the antimitotic COLCHICINE

Several currently used drugs unwantedly interfere with the synthesis of hemoglobin and thus lead to an accumulation of porphyrin in the liver and in other body organs. The authors describe an in vitro system to examine such porphyrinogenic substances. Tissues of murine liver, skin, kidneys, brain, and heart are used for explant cultures. The explants are incubated in a suitable medium for 24 hr, and the viability of the cells is controlled by measuring the release of lactate dehydrogenase (LDH) out of the cells. The studies show that porphyrinogenic drugs such as ALLYL ISOPROPYLACET-AMIDE (AIA) and VERONAL induce a considerable increase in porphyrin (measured fluorometrically) in the course of these 24 hr. The effect of AIA can be prevented or reversed in hepatocytes by adding colchicine. These studies indicate that prevailing animal experiments for the detection and closer examination of the mechanism of porphyrinogenic substances can be replaced by the presented in vitro system. Further studies on this matter are appropriate.

Type of research	basic research, applied research
Special field	pharmacology
Subject of the study	metabolism, dynamics
Target organ	heart, liver, skin, nervous system, kidney
Type of method	cell culture

Endpoint of the method	porphyrin concentration, secretion of LDH

Special characterization	psychopharmacological agents, hypnotics, soporifics, porphyrin, side effects, explant culture

Figure 9-2. Example of an entry into the databank (translated into English).

– type of research (basic, applied, etc.);
– special field (pharmacology, endocrinology, etc.);
– subject of the study (toxicity, antibody production etc.);
– target organ (heart, liver, etc.);
– method used (cell culture, computer simulation, etc.).

A number of key words are associated with each of the five key word groups. The key words were designed while working with the documents and are changed or extended according to need.

Further information on a publication includes the *endpoint* of the method. In the example, the porphyrine concentration provides information on the severity of the side effects to be expected from a specific drug. The secretion of lactate dehydrogenase (LDH) is added, because it was measured for the control of the viability of the cells.

The field *special characterization* contains specific descriptors that allow the identification of publications on similar subjects.

Practical information includes the address of the author, enabling users to contact the respective scientists, and the call number, indicating whether the publication is available in the library of the Academy for the Protection of Animals. There is also internal information giving the date when the document record was entered and a critical evaluation of the publication.

9.3   Use of the databank

There are three different possibilities of searching for information: a) The quickest method is to search for the author and/or the year of publication. b) Searching with the help of key words, chosen and combined from the thesaurus groups, selects similar studies with generally interrelated subjects. c) When performing a "full text" literature search, all entries of the databank, or certain fields of each entry, such as the summary or the special characterization, are scanned for any given word. Thus the full text search provides the possibility of doing a literature search on specific subjects. Depending on the inquiry, a broad or narrow spectrum of information is obtained.

9.4   Conclusion

The databank for alternatives to animal experiments is conceived as an informational basis for promoting the reduction and, as the final goal, the replacement of animal experiments. Thus the results of a literature search done with the help of the databank on any given subject are provided free of charge to anyone who would like to gather information about alternatives to animal experiments. Users of the databank include scientists, public authorities, and animal rightists.

The German Animal Welfare Act states that animal experiments may be performed only if they have been approved by the responsible authority and only if the scientist can prove that the objectives of the experiment cannot be achieved by in vitro methods. Therefore the databank is used by people who write, review, and approve applications for animal experiments. In order to facilitate access to the information in the databank, excerpts are published at regular intervals as the *Gelbe Liste* ("Yellow List") and distributed to all university libraries in Germany. In some of these libraries the PC-based database has been installed, offering scientists direct access.

Future plans include the translation of the databank into English, thus extending the availability of our information on alternatives to animal experiments to scientists from non-German-speaking countries.

10 The SIAT Research, Teaching and Consulting Program in the Area of in Vitro Toxicology. Experimental Research, Screening and Validation

Christoph A. Reinhardt

Summary

The objectives and activities of the Swiss Institute for Alternatives to Animal Testing, SIAT, are focused on research, education, and providing consultation in the field of alternatives to animal testing according to the Three Rs (Refine, Reduce, Replace). Practical courses, workshops and lectures are offered at the university level, in cooperation with the Swiss Federal Institute of Technology (ETH) and the University of Zurich. Documentation and consulting is provided in the areas of toxicology, biotechnology, human and veterinary medicine, ecology and bioethics.

The *In Vitro Toxicology Group* has put its main emphasis on neurodevelopmental research. Brain and retinal cells from chick embryos and from adult bovine brain are used as "robust" in vitro models including a blood-brain-barrier system for teratology and neurotoxicology. Morphology, cytotoxicity and differentiation markers of nerve, glial and endothelial cells are monitored to predict cell toxicity of drugs and chemicals. A new screening system "CHEN" (chick embryo neural cell system) is presented, which is recommended for an early screening phase in product development covering neuroteratological adverse effects. CHEN, combined with the blood-brain-barrier model and other in vitro assays, can lead to a substantial reduction of whole animal testing in screening and risk assessment.

Abbreviations. CHEN = chick embryo neural cell system; DIV = days in vitro; ED = embryonic day; ERGATT = European Research Group for Alternatives in Toxicity Testing; GFAP = glial fibrillary acidic protein; MBP = myelin basic protein; MPTP = 1-methyl-4-phenyl-1,2,3,6-tetrahydropyridine; NF = neurofilament protein; TH = tyrosine hydroxylase; SIAT = Swiss Institute for Alternatives to Animal Testing.

10.1 Introduction

When the Swiss Institute for Alternatives to Animal Testing (SIAT) was established in 1990, its founders – a group of seven dedicated individuals – conceived SIAT as an institute providing research, education, and consultation in the field of alternatives to animal testing according to the Three Rs (Refine, Reduce, Replace). The institute SIAT is supervised and financially supported by the Foundation SIAT, which is controlled by the Swiss government

Alternatives to Animal Testing. New Ways in the Biomedical Sciences, Trends and Progress.
Reinhardt, C. A. (ed.). 1994. © VCH, Weinheim.

(Figure 10-1). Most of the 26 councillors of the Foundation have an academic background in biomedicine, veterinary medicine, chemistry or in the philosophical sciences. Some of the councillors represent private organizations such as Swiss animal protection groups, the Swiss pharmaceutical industry, and a management company. Three councillors are members of Swiss or German regulatory authorities, and four are active members of the Swiss Parliament, representing different political parties. Therefore, SIAT constitutes an alliance representing ethical interests, regulatory concerns, academia and the applied biomedical sciences, where animal-based research and testing is relevant. In its research activities, SIAT focuses on toxicology and pharmacology, two fields in which the majority of seriously discomforting animal testing is performed world wide.

The institute currently consists of two research groups: The *In Vitro Toxicology Group* is installed at Technopark, Zurich, which is also the domicile of the foundation and the secretariat. The *Computer-Assisted Drug Design (CADD) Group*, operates from a facility in Basel (Vedani, 1994, this volume). The research activities at the SIAT are secured by equipment

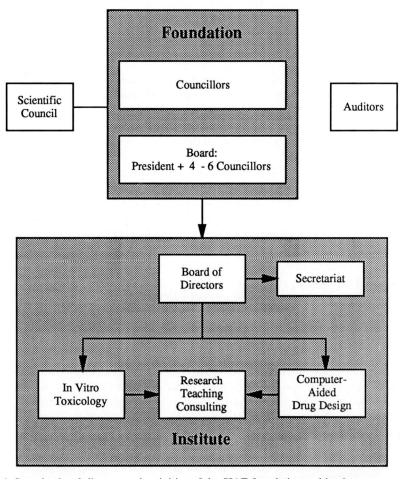

Figure 10-1. Organizational diagram and activities of the SIAT foundation and institute.

purchased with foundation funds. Individual research projects are supported by external funding (Swiss National Science Foundation, the Swiss government, industry, private organizations, the European Community). Commissioned research in the fields of in vitro toxicology and CADD supports the activities of the institute.

10.2   The need for educational programs and consulting

Recently, the Swiss animal protection law has been revised (Tierschutzgesetz, 1991) to include a paragraph which provides for the establishment of a federal bureau of documentation for alternatives to animal testing. In cooperation with this bureau, the SIAT offers practical courses, workshops and lectures for students in biology, human and veterinary medicine, ecology, philosophy, and bioethics. In this way, potential users of laboratory animals have the opportunity, already in the planning phase, to explore and evaluate the possibilities and limitations of alternative techniques to animal testing in their field. Furthermore, in most laboratory animal units, training courses in the handling of animals are now offered in compliance with the legal requirement that stressful conditions for animals before, during and after an experiment be reduced.

However, in Switzerland there is no formal prerequisite to be fulfilled and no compulsory course, as, for example, in the Netherlands (see van Zutphen, 1994, this volume), to be taken before a scientist can perform an animal experiment. Moreover, literature surveys on possible alternatives are not formally requested in the application procedure for animal experimentation, although it is conceivable that the well-functioning ZEBET literature service could be used for such purposes (see Spielmann *et al.*, 1994, this volume).

Educational programs on alternatives to animal testing are still rare in biomedicine and the related experimental sciences. Recently, I cooperated in the introduction of a new curriculum at the Department of Environmental Sciences of the Swiss Federal Institute of Technology, which emphasizes treating laboratory animals – together with farm and other domesticated animals – as our cultural partners (Reinhardt, 1993a). However, this educational program called "Environmental Hygiene" still awaits implementation in new or reorganized research units. In various other countries, efforts are now being made to set up similar educational programs specifically aimed at the concept of the Three Rs (Červinka *et al.*, 1994, this volume).

Consulting on validation and specific methodologies is offered by SIAT for carrying out intra- and interlaboratory programs (Balls *et al.*, 1990a). This is needed because such programs tend to become extremely time- and labor-intensive. Implementation and acceptance of alternatives by regulatory authorities can also be accelerated if competent consultation is sought (Balls *et al.*, 1990b). A close and coordinated collaboration with appropriate national and international organizations is essential if this goal is to be reached. Therefore SIAT works together not only with the already mentioned alternatives documentation bureau at the Swiss Federal Veterinary Office (Bern), but also with ZEBET (Berlin), FRAME (Nottingham), and the newly established European center ECVAM (Ispra), as well as with EC and OECD regulatory bodies and various laboratories within the pharmaceutical industry. Moreover, the Swiss branch of the international databank INVITTOX (*In Vitro* Techniques in Toxicology) of the European Research Group for Alternatives in Toxicity Testing (ERGATT) is located at SIAT in Zurich.

Individual consulting activity is still the most efficient way to introduce alternative techniques for routine applications. The service offered by SIAT includes specific expert recommendations on methods, validation status, and software development.

10.3   Goal of the SIAT In Vitro Toxicology Group

The *In Vitro Toxicology Group* is located at Technopark Zurich, a newly established applied research center with a large infrastructure allowing an optimal synergy between research groups of the ETH Zurich and small pioneer companies, for which the combination of production areas with the corresponding managerial and organizational support is ideal. The SIAT In Vitro Toxicology Group has recently set up a fully equipped cell laboratory, and started its activities in research, education and consulting at the Technopark in July 1993.

The general goal of the *In Vitro Toxicology Group* is the development, validation and implementation of cellular systems as alternatives to animal experiments. Selected cell systems are used for the screening of potentially harmless chemicals during product development as well as for mandatory regulatory purposes in the process of risk assessment and the registration of new products. Various ongoing validation studies for new cellular test systems, e. g. to replace the rabbit skin and eye irritation tests (see Balls and Fentem, 1994, this volume; Spielmann *et al.*, 1994, this volume), have led to the conclusion that the predictive relevance of *some* of these new systems has already been accepted by regulatory authorities. A growing number of companies is now moving into the in vitro market, which might become a major factor in the huge biotechnology market sector as in vitro technology advances (see e. g. Danheiser, 1993). SIAT also offers services including consultation and commissioned testing for promising in vitro models.

For other areas of toxicology (such as teratology, neurotoxicology, organ-specific toxicology and carcinogenesis), in vitro models – as well as many of the in vivo models in use – have rarely been validated. An update of the first Amden workshop on validation (Balls *et al.*, 1990a) is planned by ERGATT in early 1994 to develop a scientific framework for manageable validation procedures and to find practical ways of implementing validated tests. Relevant in vitro models still need to be developed, c. g. for screening potentially harmless drugs and chemicals within selected groups of pharmacologically active molecules. Thus, a strong engagement in research and a close collaboration with toxicologists and pharmacologists in industrial laboratories is crucial at this stage of the development of alternatives.

10.4   The research program of the SIAT In Vitro Toxicology Group

10.4.1   In vitro neuroteratology
The interrelationship between the teratogenicity and neurotoxicity of bioreactive agents is still largely unknown, although a large background of neurobiological and developmental research at the cellular level is available, e. g. for glial-neuronal interactions (Abbott, 1991). Since most teratogenic chemicals primarily affect the nervous system, an in vitro short-term assay to screen for potential teratogens would preferentially need to include differentiating and functional neural cells in culture. Embryonic cells from whole brain and retina tissues were therefore selected at a stage in which cell isolation is routinely manageable and in which

differentiation has just begun. The chick has been selected in order to avoid the unnecessary killing of a mother animal (as in the case of all mammalian embryo work) and because the most sensitive developmental stage of the embryo can be easily and reproducibly selected. Three culture methods are used: a) monolayer cultures for short treatment periods (up to 7 days), b) aggregated cell cultures (reaggregates) under constant gyratory movement for treatment periods up to several months, and c) 14-day-old reaggregates attached to petri dish or glass surfaces for short treatments of already stably differentiated neural cells. Morphology, cytotoxicity and differentiation of nerve and glial cells in brain and retina are monitored: neurofilament (NF) and microtubule-associated proteins (nerve cells), glial fibrillary acidic protein (GFAP, astrocytes) and myelin basic protein (MBP, oligodendrocytes). All these markers seem to develop in time periods comparable to those known from the in vivo development, except that GFAP is expressed earlier and stronger than in the corresponding tissue left in the embryo (Table 10-1).

Table 10-1. Comparison of the expression of cellular differentiation markers in the normal chick embryo (in vivo) and in reaggregates of embryonic chick brain cells (in vitro) (Wyle, 1992; Wyle and Reinhardt, 1991)

	In vitro ED7 cells 7 DIV	In vivo ED14
Nerve cells		
NF staining in all cells	+++	+++
TH staining in single cells	+++	+++
Astrocytes		
GFAP staining	+++	+
Oligodendrocytes		
MBP staining	–	–

DIV = days in vitro
ED = embryonic day

10.4.2   CHEN, the chick embryo neural cell assay

Validation of the chick embryo neural cell assay has been done with a series of 16 known neuroteratogens and non-teratogens using coded test chemicals (Reinhardt, 1993b). In conjunction with the ECITTS project, an interlaboratory validation program has been started (Walum *et al.*, 1992). With this project, it is also anticipated to be able to reduce or even replace some of the animal tests in behavioral teratology which are notoriously unreliable because of their low sensitivity and low specificity (Francis, 1992).

Reaggregate cultures develop in a few days from randomly adhering cell clusters into solid, round reaggregates. After one week they often show several growth cones, which smooth out into perfect spheres after another week and are then stable in size for several months.

Nerve cells already show positive staining for NF from the onset of the cultures. Long and elaborate neurites form in a few days, which accumulate particularly in the outer layer of the reaggregates (Figure 10-2a).

Astrocytes of type 2 stain positive for GFAP. Stained cells appear in small clusters after three days in cultured reaggregates. After two weeks they are abundant throughout the entire

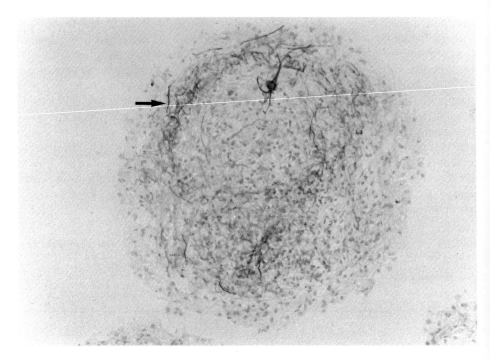

a

b

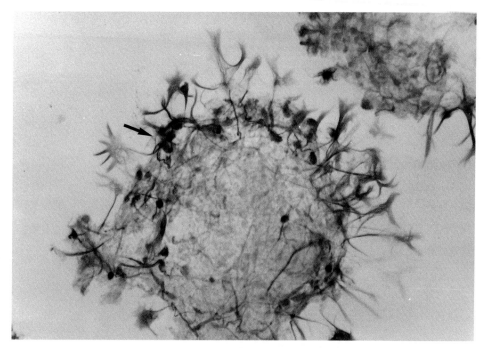

c

Figure 10-2. Chick embryonic brain cell reaggregates used for the chick embryo neurotoxicity (CHEN) assay. a) Frozen section through a 14-DIV cultured brain cell reaggregate, immunocytochemical PAP stain for 68-kD neurofilament (arrow). b) Phase contrast view and c) bright light view of a whole mount re-aggregate (14 DIV plus 3 days reattached to glass), immunocytochemical PAP stain for GFAP (arrow).

reaggregates (Figure 10-2b). Thus, in contrast to NF, GFAP is not expressed at the start of the cultures but fully develops in vitro within a few days. Therefore, GFAP could serve as a marker to trace any changes in the development of astrocytes in vitro.

The detailed protocol of the CHEN assay is registered at the INVITTOX methodology databank. In short, the procedure uses routine, purchasable, cell culture and immunocyto-chemistry materials. Serum-free medium is used after an initial one-week aggregation forming phase. The treatment procedure is divided into two periods: a) 0–14 days in vitro (DIV) to monitor the differentiation processes, and b) 14–17 DIV to monitor neurotoxic effects in differentiated reaggregates. Interpretation of the results is based on the ELISA microassay and on the evaluation of morphological immunostaining (Sternberger, 1986) of the differentiation and functional neural markers.

The CHEN assay can also be used for monitoring specific neurotoxicological effects of chemicals. The dopaminergic system is monitored by measuring transmitter synthesis and release as well as by determining the activity of the key enzyme tyrosine hydroxylase (TH). The in vitro effects of well-known neurotoxins and behavior-affecting drugs (such as 1-methyl-4-phenyl-1,2,3,6-tetrahydropyridine (MPTP) and heavy metals) and of various chemicals (such as pesticides and herbicides) show that the relevance of the system is promising when comparing the in vitro effects with animal toxicity profiles and particularly with effects on humans (for examples see Table 10-2).

Table 10-2. Comparison of lowest effect levels (LOEL) in vitro and in vivo for four potential neurotoxins

Test substance	In vitro Chick cells LOEL	In vitro Rat cells LOEL	In vivo Human Toxic plasma level
Cadmium chloride	<0.87 μM^a 0.55 μM^d	<5.5 μM^b	0.055 μM^c
Cytarabinoside (Ara-C)	0.40 μM^a	<0.36 μM^b 0.4 μM^f	0.036–0.54 μM^e
Diphenylhydantoin (phenytoin)	15.0 μM^a 300.0 μM^d	100.0 μM^b 80.0 μM^f	79.0 μM^g
MPTP	1.0 μM^a	0.1 μM^h	1.0 μM^i

[a] CHEN assays (14-DIV reaggregates treated 3d in vitro) (this study).
[b] Micromass rat midbrain cell culture according to Flint and Orton (1984).
[c] Carmichael *et al.* (1982).
[d] CERC, Chick Embryo Neural Retina Cell assay according to Daston *et al.* (1991).
[e] Morant and Ruppanner (1990).
[f] Reaggregated rat brain cells according to Honegger and Werffeli (1988).
[g] Plaa (1975).
[h] Tyrosine immunoreactivity in fetal rat cells according to Sanchez-Ramoz *et al.* (1988).
[i] Data for the active metabolite MPP+ in monkey brain tissue according to Yang *et al.* (1988).

10.4.3 Blood-brain barrier in vitro

A new blood-brain-barrier model based on bovine brain tissue from a local slaughterhouse (Miller and Borchardt, 1991; Rubin *et al.*, 1991) will be used in combination with the neuro-teratolgy assay in vitro and the CHEN assays (see above). Freshly isolated brain endothelial cells are reconstituted to an intact endothelium on an artificial membrane by adding astrocyte-conditioned serum-free medium to the forming monolayer. Barrier and transport functions of this in vitro blood-brain-barrier model are monitored upon treatment with test chemicals. This will allow us to improve the predictive power for the determination of neurotoxic potential on a purely in vitro basis.

10.4.4 New projects

A further project deals with the replacement of OECD guidelines 418 and 419 on delayed neurotoxicity testing of organophosphorous substances. According to these guidelines, acute and repeated doses of organophosphates have to be given to adult hens, which then develop ataxia and other clinical signs of neuropathy very similar to those in humans (Lotti, 1991). Hens and humans also develop an early marker protein, neuropathy target esterase (or neurotoxic esterase, NTE), which can also be induced in primary cultures and in some cell lines (Johnson, 1990; Nostrandt and Ehrich, 1992). The use and validation of the NTE assay will be studied and a robust protocol developed.

In addition, cellular stress is being studied with modern biotechnology tools, such as northern blotting, to monitor stress protein regulation, RNAase, and RNA regulation during culture adaptation of primary neural cells such as activated astrocytes.

10.5 Outlook

A battery of cell systems would have to be developed in order to determine the toxic levels in the most important target tissues, on the basis of which the toxic potential in man could be predicted without using live animals. Ongoing projects are aimed at a) improving the application of lipophilic drugs and chemicals to monolayer cultures and reaggregation cultures, and b) developing new reaggregation culture systems from adult tissue of various organs.

Robust bioassays are needed that can easily be used by routine laboratories to build up a large database – the most important prerequisite for successful validation and acceptance by regulatory authorities (Balls *et al.*, 1990a, 1990b).

Although it must be acknowledged that only part of the biokinetic behavior of a potential neurotoxin can be modelled with any of the mentioned assays, we are confident that an intelligent combination of all test results holds future promise for a predictive in vitro toxicology.

Acknowledgements. This work has been supported by the Foundation Swiss Institute for Alternatives to Animal Testing (SIAT), Zurich and by a grant from the Roche Research Foundation, Basel.

References

Abbott N. J. (Editor) (1991) Glial-neuronal interaction. *Annals of the New York Academy of Sciences* **633,** 639 pp.

Balls M., Blaauboer B., Brusick D., Frazier J., Lamb D., Pemberton M., Reinhardt C., Roberfroid M., Rosenkranz H., Schmid B., Spielmann H., Stammati A.-L. and Walum E. (1990a) Report and recommendations of the CAAT/ERGATT workshop on the validation of toxicity test procedures. *ATLA* **18,** 313–337.

Balls M., Botham P., Cordier A., Fumero S., Kayser D., Koëter H., Koundakjian P., Lindquist N. G., Meyer O., Pioda L., Reinhardt C., Rozemond H., Smyrniotis T., Spielmann H., Van Looy H., van der Venne M.-T. and Walum E. (1990b) Report and recommendations of an international workshop on promotion of the regulatory acceptance of validated non-animal toxicity test procedures. *ATLA* **18,** 339–344.

Balls M. and Fentem J. H. (1994) The Fund for the Replacement of Animals in Medical Experiments (FRAME): 23 years of campaigning for the Three Rs. In *Alternatives to Animal Testing. New Ways in the Biomedical Sciences, Trends and Progress.* Edited by C. A. Reinhardt. pp. 45–55. VCH Verlagsgesellschaft, Weinheim.

Carmichael N. G., Backhouse B. L., Winder C. and Lewis P. D. (1982) Teratogenicity, toxicity and perinatal effect of cadmium. *Human Toxicology* **1,** 159–186.

Červinka M., Červinkova Z., Balls M. and Spielmann H. (1994) Alternatives to experiments with animals in medical education: A TEMPUS Joint European Project. In *Alternatives to Animal Testing. New Ways in the Biomedical Sciences, Trends and Progress.* Edited by C. A. Reinhardt. pp. 119–123. VCH Verlagsgesellschaft, Weinheim.

Danheiser S. L. (1993) In vitro test alternatives market faces growth obstacles as technology advances. *Genetic Engineering News* **13,** 1, 3, 5, 20.

Daston G. P., Baines D. and Yonker J. E. (1991) Chick embryo neural retina cell culture as a screen for developmental toxicity. *Toxicology and Applied Pharmacology* **109,** 352–366.

Flint O. P. and Orton T. C. (1984) An in vitro assay for teratogens with cultures of rat embryo midbrain and limb bud cells. *Toxicology and Applied Pharmacology* **76,** 383–395.

Francis E. Z. (1992) Regulatory developmental neurotoxicity and human risk assessment. *NeuroToxicology* **13,** 77–84.

Honegger P. and Werffeli P. (1988) Use of aggregating cell cultures for toxicological studies. *Experientia* **44**, 817–822.

Johnson M. K. (1990) Contemporary issues in toxicology. Organophosphates and delayed neuropathy – is NTE alive and well? *Toxicology and Applied Pharmacology* **102**, 385–399.

Lotti M. (1991) The pathogenesis of organophosphate polyneuropathy. *Critical Reviews in Toxicology* **21**, 465–487.

Miller D. W. and Borchardt R. T. (1991) Distribution of insulin binding sites on cultured bovine brain endothelial cells and their possible role in the transport of insulin across the blood-brain barrier. *Journal of Neuroscience* **45**, 236 (Abstract 1512).

Morant J. and Ruppanner H. (Editors) (1990) *Arzneimittel-Kompendium der Schweiz* (12th ed.). p. 99. Documed AG, Basel.

Nostrandt A. C. and Ehrich M. (1992) Development of a model cell culture system in which to study early effects of neuropathy-inducing organophosphorus esters. *Toxicology Letters* **60**, 107–114.

Plaa G. L. (1975) Acute toxicity of antiepileptic drugs. *Epilepsia* **16**, 183–191.

Reinhardt C. A. (1993a) Alternativen zu Tierversuchen als Lehrfach: Für neue Wege in den biomedizinischen Wissenschaften. In *Tierschutz durch Alternativen*. Edited by W. Hardegg, I. Livaditis and M. Vogt. pp. 226–234. Verlag Gesundheit, Berlin.

Reinhardt C. A. (1993b) Neurodevelopmental toxicity in vitro. *Reproductive Toxicology* **7**, 165–170.

Rubin L. L., Hall D. E., Porter S., Barbu K., Cannon C., Horner H. C., Janatpour M., Liaw C. W., Manning K., Morales J., Tanner L. I., Tomaselli K. J. and Bard F. (1991) A cell culture model of the blood-brain barrier. *Journal of Cell Biology* **115**, 1725–1735.

Sanchez-Ramoz J. R, Michel P., Weiner W. J. and Hefti F. (1988) Selective destruction of cultured dopaminergic neurons from fetal rat mesencephalon by 1-methyl-4-phenyl-tetrahydropyridine: Cytochemical and morphological evidence. *Journal of Neurochemistry* **50**, 1934–1944.

Spielmann H., Grune-Wolff B. and Liebsch M. (1994) ZEBET: Three years of the National German Center for Documentation and Evaluation of Alternatives to Animal Experiments at the Federal Health Office (BGA) in Berlin. In *Alternatives to Animal Testing. New Ways in the Biomedical Sciences, Trends and Progress*. Edited by C. A. Reinhardt. pp. 75–84. VCH Verlagsgesellschaft, Weinheim.

Sternberger L. A. (1986) The unlabeled antibody peroxidase (PA) method. Staining for light microscopy. In *Immunocytochemistry*. Edited by L. A. Sternberger. pp. 103–114. John Wiley, New York.

Tierschutzgesetz (1991) Änderung vom 22. März 1991. AS 1991 2345–2348; *Bundesblatt III,* 1257.

van Zutphen L. F. M. (1994) Animal use and alternatives: Developments in the Netherlands. In *Alternatives to Animal Testing. New Ways in the Biomedical Sciences, Trends and Progress*. Edited by C. A. Reinhardt. pp. 57–65. VCH Verlagsgesellschaft, Weinheim.

Vedani A. (1994) Computer-aided drug design and the Three Rs. In *Alternatives to Animal Testing. New Ways in the Biomedical Sciences, Trends and Progress*. Edited by C. A. Reinhardt. pp. 99–106. VCH Verlagsgesellschaft, Weinheim.

Walum E., Balls M., Bianchi V., Blaauboer B., Bolcsfoldi G., Guillouzo A., Moore G. A., Odland L., Reinhardt C. A. and Spielmann H. (1992) ECITTS: An integrated approach to the application of in vitro test systems to the hazard assessment of chemicals. *ATLA* **20**, 406–428.

Wyle-Gyurech G. G. (1992) *Embryonic chick brain cells as a potential model for developmental toxicity: An immunocytochemical study*. Doctoral dissertation Nr. 9677, ETH Zurich.

Wyle-Gyurech G. G. and Reinhardt C. A. (1991) In vitro differentiation of embryonic chick brain cells: Development of a neurotoxicity test system. *Toxicology in Vitro* **6**, 419–425.

Yang S. C., Johannessen J. N. and Markey S. P. (1988) Metabolism of (^{14}C) MPTP in mouse and monkey implicates MPP$^+$, and not bound metabolites, as the operative neurotoxin. *Chemical Research and Toxicology* **1**, 228–233.

11   Computer-Aided Drug Design and the Three Rs

Angelo Vedani

Summary

Computer-aided drug design (CADD) permits the screening of large series of molecules for potential pharmacological activity without having to synthesize the chemical beforehand and apply it to in vitro or in vivo systems. Instead, the pharmacological activity of a molecule can be assessed by generating its molecular structure in a computer and simulating its interaction with the target receptor. Specifically, a newly developed computer program using the technique of *pseudereceptor modeling* is described together with the results of its validation using the enzyme carbonic anhydrase. Computer-based screening techniques have a potential for significantly reducing animal testing compared with the classical approaches to drug discovery, as weakly binding drugs or inactive drugs can be recognized at an early stage and thus removed from the evaluation process before in vivo testing is involved.

11.1   Introduction

The philosophy of computer-aided drug design (CADD) is based on the lock-and-key analogy, recognized as early as 1894 by the German chemist and Nobel laureate, Emil Fischer. According to this analogy, a natural (or synthetic) drug fits into a biological receptor like a mechanical key fits into a mechanical lock. The drug might, therefore, be referred to as a *biological key*, the receptor as the *biological lock*.

In contrast to a mechanical key, a biological key displays a far more complex structure: composition, size, shape, electric, and electronic properties are responsible for its activity, or inactivity. Most important, a biological key is a highly flexible structure. Its interaction with the environment (recognition, binding, chemical reactivity) must be understood as a dynamic process, rather than as a rigid lock-and-key scheme. The dynamics of molecules can be simulated with a computer; knowledge of the dynamic behavior of both lock and key is a prerequisite for any drug-design study.

Of course, the biological lock is also a dynamic structure and can, therefore, adapt its shape to a biological key as well (induced-fit mechanism). Complexity and flexibility of drug and receptor are responsible for a vast number of combinations. Their simulation in CADD applications requires powerful computers and computer-graphics systems. By simulating

Alternatives to Animal Testing. New Ways in the Biomedical Sciences, Trends and Progress.
Reinhardt, C. A. (ed.). 1994. © VCH, Weinheim.

and analyzing the most likely structural combinations of lock and key, CADD is a tool for developing taylor-made drug molecules.

The advantages of CADD in comparison with classical approaches to drug discovery are twofold: Firstly, CADD permits the screening of a large series of molecules for a potential pharmacological activity without having to synthesize the chemical beforehand, i. e. the pharmacological activity of a molecule can be assessed by generating its molecular structure in a computer and simulating its interaction with the target receptor. Secondly, and most important for the aims of the SIAT, CADD is a screening technique with a significant potential for reducing animal testing. The recognition of weakly binding or inactive drugs at a very early stage allows the removal of these compounds from the evaluation process before in vivo testing is involved. In industrial applications, over 90 % of the screened compounds are eliminated in this first pass; if the screening method is in vitro or "in computo," the benefit for the Three Rs is maximal.

11.2   Methods

CADD comprises various techniques aimed at identifying pharmacologically potent molecules by means of numerical and graphical simulation (Burgen *et al.*, 1986; Cohen *et al.*, 1990; Fauchere, 1989; Hadzi and Jerman-Blazic, 1987; Perun and Probst, 1989; Ramsden, 1990; Rein and Golombek, 1989; van der Goot, 1989; van Gunsteren and Weiner, 1989; Vida and Gordon, 1984). If the three-dimensional structure of the receptor is available, a technique referred to as *receptor-fitting* allows the identification of structural properties of potential drug molecules for a given receptor. Using the terminology of the lock-and-key analogy, CADD allows the identification of an optimal biological key for a given biological lock.

For practical purposes, one generally starts with the *natural key* (the substrate) of the receptor and then proceeds to employ minor or major chemical modifications in the computer until a molecule with the desired properties is identified. A potent drug molecule should mimic the natural substrate but include additional structural elements (functional groups) to achieve a selective binding. Apart from cytostatics, interactions between drug and receptor should be non-covalent in character, as the benefits of the drug should vanish after removal from therapy. In a final step, those molecules identified as potentially active by means of CADD are synthesized and tested for activity using in vitro or in vivo methods.

Unfortunately, a detailed three-dimensional structure is only available for a few receptors of medicinal interest, presently some 50 to 100. For all other systems, receptor-fitting would not seem to be directly applicable.

As an approach to this problem, a technique termed *receptor mapping* has been devised in the last decade (Hibert, 1990; Ramsden, 1990). Its principle is simple: By superimposing bioactive compounds (drug molecules), known to bind to the structurally uncharacterized receptor, it should be possible to recognize features essential for binding, and, subsequently, to taylor an optimal drug molecule. So far, this technique has not reached the accuracy of receptor fitting, and never will, as the detailed three-dimensional structure of the receptor remains unknown. As a consequence, the potential for reducing animal testing by means of receptor mapping is limited.

Missing from the molecular design toolkit is a means for linking the two approaches: a technique for performing receptor fitting in a receptor-mapping context. A comprehensive strategy for combining receptor fitting and receptor mapping is the construction of a pseudoreceptor, an explicit molecular binding pocket for a series of molecules, known to bind to a particular receptor (Snyder *et al.*, 1992). In other words, pseudoreceptor modeling attempts to reconstruct a receptor, based on the structure of already known bioactive molecules. In a subsequent step, the best receptor model is used to taylor an even better drug.

In cooperation with a Chicago-based pharmaceutical company, we have developed the computer program Yak© (Snyder *et al.*, in press; Vedani *et al.*, 1993), named after this most amiable species living in the high Himalayas. The program allows the explicit construction of a peptide receptor around a single molecule or any molecular ensemble of interest.

The mapping process in Yak is based on a concept known as *directionality of molecular interactions* (see, for example, Alexander *et al.*, 1990; Baker and Hubbard, 1984; Murray-Rust and Glusker, 1984; Taylor and Kennard, 1984; Tintelnot and Andrews, 1989; Vedani and Dunitz, 1985), i.e. each part of a natural or synthetic drug has very distinct preferences for how it can favorably interact with a receptor. In Yak, such preferences are represented as vectors. If a set of superimposed molecules is analyzed, we assume that portions of Cartesian space where these vectors cluster, indicate possibly important interaction sites on the receptor. A cluster analysis reveals which functional groups of the used molecules are relevant for interacting with the receptor.

Next, a *preference database*, compiled from data retrieved from the Brookhaven Protein Data Bank (Bernstein *et al.*, 1977), suggests the most probable amino-acid residue to interact with a given functional group of the drug molecule. Then, the amino-acid residue (or a metal-ion template) is retrieved from a structural database, aligned, oriented, and energy optimized. The set of amino acids in the residue database represents the Ponder-Richards side-chain rotamer library (Ponder and Richards, 1987). This process is repeated until all functional groups are saturated, or, alternatively, until spatial requirements forbid the further attachment of residues. The ultimate goal of the program is to generate a pseudoreceptor to which the known bioactive molecules bind in the same relative strength as they do towards the true biological receptor.

The Yak force field represents the all-atom version of the Yeti© force field (Vedani and Huhta, 1990), their minimizers are identical. The solvation routine of Yak is based on the Yeti module AUTO–SOL (Vedani and Huhta, 1991). The program is fully interactive, menu-driven, and includes a graphics shell allowing for real-time three-dimensional visualization of the mapping process. On-line help is available throughout the mapping process. The flow chart of the program is shown in Figure 11-1.

11.3   Validation

To test the concept of Yak, we have performed several simulations aimed at reproducing the binding site of two known proteins, carbonic anhydrase and thermolysin. Results on carbonic anhydrase are discussed below: based on the structures of four sulfonamide inhibitor molecules, a series of models were generated for the active site of the enzyme. The best model deviates by 1.7 Å from the experimentally determined structure; for the six most relevant interaction sites the deviation is as small as 0.7 Å. Details are given in Table 11-1 and shown in Figure 11-2.

The catalytic zinc (Zn^{2+}) was reproduced best, located only 0.156 Å off the X-ray position. The three zinc-bound imidazole residues (representing histidine residues in Yak) are

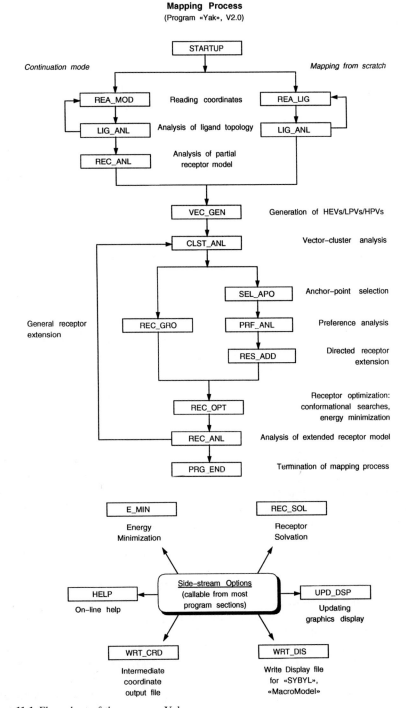

Figure 11-1. Flow chart of the program Yak.

Table 11-1. Comparison of key atomic positions of a model for carbonic anhydrase I as generated by Yak with the X-ray crystal structure of the native enzyme. A) Metal-binding site; B) Upper, hydrophilic part of the active-site cleft; C) Lower, hydrophobic part of the active-site cleft.

	X-ray data		Yak model			
	Residue	Atom	Residue	Atom	Offset	Orientation
A)	Het	Zn(II)	Het	Zn(II)	0.156 Å	–
	His 94	NE2	Imi[a]	NB	0.427 Å	ring rotated 75°
	His 96	NE2	Imi[a]	NB	0.297 Å	correct
	His 119	ND1	Imi[a]	NB	0.244 Å	ring rotated 45°
B)	Leu 198	CG	Leu	CG	2.054 Å	slightly rotated
		CD1		CD1	2.906 Å	
		CD2		CD2	2.676 Å	
	Thr 199	H	Ser[b]	H	1.481 Å	correct
		OG1		OG	1.472 Å	
C)	Phe 91	CZ	Phe	CZ	1.806 Å	correct
		CE2		CE2	1.683 Å	
	Gln 92	OE1	Gln	OE1	1.986 Å	side chain
		HNE1		HNE1	3.332 Å	slightly rotated
	Leu 131	CD2	Leu	CD2	2.983 Å	side chain correct

[a] Zinc-bound imidazole residue as Yak template; corresponding atomic positions are compared.
[b] Serine residue in Yak receptor model (native: Thr); corresponding atomic positions are compared.
| = residues linked by amide bonds.

displaced 0.427 Å, 0.297 Å, and 0.244 Å from the experimental position, respectively. As the model includes only *one shell of protein*, the orientation of the histidine rings is not reproduced perfectly. Nonetheless, the imidazole mimicking His 94 does engage in a H-bond with the side-chain amide O of residue Gln 92.

In the X-ray structure (as well as in model studies), threonine 199 is found to engage in two interactions with the sulfonamide inhibitor: a) The amide-H atom forms a hydrogen bond with the side-chain hydroxyl O. b) One sulfonamide-O atom (not coordinated to the zinc) engages in a H-bond interaction with the main-chain amide >N-H atom.

Yak preferred serine over threonine for energy reasons (although a different side-chain orientation was observed). However, both H-bond interactions are reproduced by Yak. The deviation of the hydroxyl O atom from the experimental position is 1.472 Å, the deviation of the main-chain amide H atom 1.481 Å.

In the X-ray structure, as well as in model studies (Vedani and Huhta, 1990), threonine 199 is found to engage in two interactions with the sulfonamide inhibitor: a) Its side-chain hydroxyl O atom forms a H-bond with the one of the sulfonamide-O atoms (not coordinated to the zinc). b) Its main-chain amide engages in a H-bond with the amide-H atom. In the model generated by Yak, a serine was preferred over threonine for energy reasons; however,

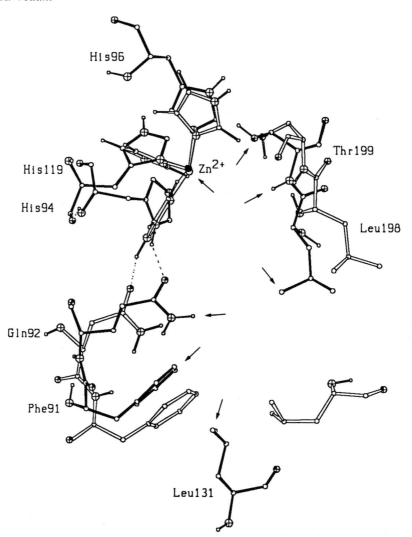

Figure 11-2. Comparison of a model for the enzyme human carbonic anhydrase I, as generated by Yak (open lines) with the X-ray crystal structure of the native enzyme (solid lines). Important interaction sites for the binding of the sulfonamide inhibitors are marked by arrows; apolar H atoms are omitted for clarity.

both interactions were reproduced. The deviation of the hydroxyl O atom in the model structure from the experimental position is 1.472 Å, the deviation of the main-chain H atom 1.481 Å.

Leucine 198 was reproduced almost perfectly, its amide bond with residue 199 formed correctly. The positions of their side-chain atoms differ by 2.906 Å (CD1; BPDB notation for carbon atom at the delta 1 position) and 2.676 Å (CD2), respectively. Overall, residues 198 and 199 are oriented correctly, but shifted appproximately 1.4 Å in their main-chain position (alpha-carbon atoms).

Residue glutamine 92 was reproduced satisfactorily: Its H-bond interactions with the ligands and the imidazole ring (mimicking His 94) are present in the model. Also, the amide bond from Phe 91 to Gln 92 was formed almost atop that of the X-ray structure. Due to the slightly different position of Imi 6 (ring rotated 75°), the side-chain of Gln 92 is shifted by about 1.02.0 Å, but otherwise (except its side-chain amide plane) oriented correctly. OE1 is 1.986 Å off the experimental position; HNE13.696 Å.

Residue phenylalanine 91 (including its amide link to Gln 92) was reproduced perfectly in the Yak model, the deviations (of CZ and CE2) from the experimental positions being 1.806 and 1.683 Å, respectively.

Residue leucine 131 is shifted approximately 2.0 Å in the Yak model, the positions of its side-chain C atoms (CD1,CD2) being 2.755 Å and 2.983 Å off the experimental position, respectively.

11.4   Outlook

To increase the efficiency of CADD with respect to reducing and replacing animal models, receptor fitting and receptor mapping must be evolved towards the parallel simulation of metabolic, pharmacokinetic, and toxicological effects. Presently, both techniques analyze "just" the binding of the potential drug towards a given (or hypothetical) receptor. Chemistry and physics on the way to the receptor and during secretion of the drug (such as metabolism, toxicity) are not yet considered. Also, the distribution of the drug in the organism (pharmacokinetics) remains excluded. A final improvement would call for the analysis of side effects, most particularly, the binding to secondary receptors.

While the latter is basically a question of the available computing power, simulation of metabolism and toxicity is a conceptually much tougher endeavour – nonetheless, the goal of the SIAT Biographics Laboratory for the future.

Acknowledgements. I wish to express my gratitude to Dr. James P. Snyder and his coworkers at G. D. Searle & Co. (Chicago) for initiating the idea of a pseudoreceptor concept and their support throughout development and validation of the software. Financial support from G. D. Searle & Co., the Foundation for Animal-Free Research (FFVFF, Zurich), and the Foundation SIAT is also gratefully acknowledged.

References

Alexander R. S., Kanyo Z. F., Chirlian L. E. and Christianson D. W. (1990) Stereochemistry of phosphate-Lewis acid interactions: Implication for nucleic acid structure and recognition. *Journal of the American Chemical Society* **112,** 933–937.

Baker E. N. and Hubbard R. E. (1984) Hydrogen bonding in globular proteins. *Progress in Biophysics & Molecular Biology* **44,** 97–179.

Bernstein F., Koetzle T. F., Williams G. J. B., Meyer E. F., Jr., Brice M. D., Rodgers J. R., Kennard O., Shimanouchi T. and Tasumi M. J. (1977) The Brookhaven Protein Data Bank. *Journal of Molecular Biology* **112,** 535.

Burgen A. S. V., Roberts G. C. K. and Tute M. S. (Editors) (1986) *Topics in Molecular Pharmacology, Vol. 3. Molecular Graphics and Drug Design.* Elsevier, Amsterdam.

Cohen N. C., Blaney J. M., Humblet C., Gund P. and Barry D. C. (1990) Molecular modeling software and methods for medicinal chemistry. *Journal of Medicinal Chemistry* **33**, 883–894.

Fauchere J. L. (Editor) (1989) QSAR: Quantitative structure-activity relationships in drug design [Proceedings of the 7th European Symposium on QSAR]. *Progress in Clinical and Biological Research* **291**.

Hadzi D. and Jerman-Blazic B. (Editors) (1987) QSAR in drug design and toxicology [Proceedings of the 6th European Symposium on QSAR]. *Pharmacochemistry Library*. Vol. 10. Elsevier, Amsterdam.

Hibert M. (1990) Quantitative drug design. *European Journal of Pharmacology* **183**, 180.

Murray-Rust P. and Glusker J. P. (1984) Directional hydrogen bonding to sp^2 and sp^3-hybridized oxygen atoms and its relevance to ligand-macromolecule interactions. *Journal of the American Chemical Society* **106**, 1018–1025.

Perun T. J. and C. L. Probst (Editors) (1989) *Computer-Aided Drug Design: Methods and Applications.* Dekker, New York.

Ponder J. W. and Richards F. M. (1987) Tertiary templates for proteins. *Journal of Molecular Biology* **193**, 775–791.

Ramsden C. A. (Editor) (1990) *Comprehensive Medicinal Chemistry, Vol. 4. Quantitative Drug Design.* Pergamon Press, Oxford.

Rein R. and Golombek A. (Editors) (1989) Computer-assisted modeling of receptor-ligand interactions: Theoretical aspects and applications to drug design [Proceedings of the 1988 OHOLO Conference]. *Progress in Clinical and Biological Research* **289**

Snyder J. P., Rao S. N., Koehler K. F. and Pellicciari R. (1992) Drug modeling at cell membrane receptors: The concept of pseudo-receptors. In *Trends in Receptor Research*. Edited by P. Angeli, U. Gulini and W. Quaglia. pp. 367–403. Elsevier, Amsterdam.

Snyder J. P., Rao S. N., Koehler K. F. and Vedani A. (in press) Pseudoreceptors. In *3D QSAR in Drug Design*. Edited by H. Kubinyi. ESCOM Science Publishers B. V., Leiden, NL.

Taylor R. and Kennard O. (1984) Hydrogen-bond geometry in organic crystals. *Accounts of Chemical Research* **17**, 320–326.

Tintelnot M. and Andrews P. (1989) Geometries of fuctional group interactions in enzyme-ligand complexes: Guides for receptor modelling. *Journal of Computer-Aided Design* **3**, 67–84.

van der Goot H. (Editor) (1989) *Trends in Medicinal Chemistry* [Proceedings of the 10th International Symposium on Medicinal Chemistry]. Elsevier, Amsterdam.

van Gunsteren W. F. and Weiner P. K. (Editors) (1989) *Computer Simulations in Protein Engineering and Drug Design.* ESCOM, Leiden.

Vedani A. and Dunitz J. D. (1985) Lone-pair directionality in H-bond potential functions for molecular mechanics calculations. *Journal of the American Chemical Society* **107**, 7653–7658.

Vedani A. and Huhta D. W. (1990) A new force field for modeling metalloproteins. *Journal of the American Chemical Society* **112**, 4759–4767.

Vedani A. and Huhta D. W. (1991) An algorithm for the systematic solvation of proteins based on the directionality of hydrogen bonds. *Journal of the American Chemical Society* **113**, 5860–5862.

Vedani A., Zbinden P. and Snyder J. P. (1993) Pseudo-receptor modeling: A new concept for the three-dimensional construction of receptor binding sites. *Journal of Receptor Research* **13**, 163–177.

Vida J. A. and Gordon M. (Editors) (1984) Conformationally directed drug design: Peptides and nucleic acids as templates or targets. *ACS Symposium Series* **251**.

12   Computer-Aided Programs in Biomedical Education

Richard T. Fosse

Summary

Biomedical education has traditionally made use of animals in teaching student practicals. The phenomena that are demonstrated are well-known, proven physiological and pharmacological systems. Many of the systems have been analyzed and can be expressed as mathematic algorithms. Algorithms can be used to write computer programs which, when coupled to graphic output, will give the student information similar to that derived from experiments with animals. Interactive video in the form of computer controlled laser disks is another form of education that has contributed to replacing animals in biomedical education. There is reason to believe that many traditional student exercises that previously used animals can now be replaced by computerized systems that offer as good if not better teaching quality.

12.1   Introduction

Biomedical experimentation that involves animals generates considerable interest among members of the public. It is clear when addressing this subject that there are conflicting interests among lay persons and researchers. Analysis of the use of animals reveals that it is possible to divide their usage into four generalized categories: a) animals used for testing of toxicological and other chemical effects; b) animals used for research, applied and basic; c) animals used for diagnostic purposes; and d) animals used for training and other educational purposes. In the first three categories, animals are used to investigate phenomena for which the endpoint of the investigation may not always be known and in this case, the animal is used as a part of the process of hypothesis proof or disproof. In the case of toxicological investigation, animals can be used to predict unknown chemical effects or interactions. In the case of education, however, the "research"-based foundation has already been established. The prime goal of the exercise here is to transfer previously proved and confirmed knowledge from a teacher to a student.

Broadly speaking, there are two major issues that determine the acceptability of computers as alternatives. Firstly, does the computer version have the same or similar pedagogical value as teaching methods that make use of animals, and, secondly, are there sufficient computerized systems available that cover most or all of the fields that need to be taught?

Alternatives to Animal Testing. New Ways in the Biomedical Sciences, Trends and Progress.
Reinhardt, C. A. (ed.). 1994. © VCH, Weinheim.

12.2   Pedagogical value

Medical education has two major objectives. The first of these is the provision of a broad theoretical background and the second is providing students with the practical experience needed to reinforce the theory. Biomedicine is based on an extensive experimental foundation. Much of the experimentation has been performed on animals, and the paradigms that make up much of the knowledge of the human system are in fact derived from species other than man. There are therefore several pedagogical objectives to be met when teaching biomedical students in laboratory classes. These include providing students with new and updated information and enabling them to apply this knowledge quickly and efficiently. Current established know-how should be reinforced and applied to the relevant theory base. Students should have the opportunity to attain and practice skills in experimental design and methodology. Experimental data obtained in the course of the practical training should be processed and interpreted. There should be opportunity for critical appraisal of data as well as training in the reporting and presentation of data. Students should be given the opportunity to work in teams, with fellow students and teachers. Depending on the area being studied, students should be able to train in specific laboratory skills.

It is clear that all these elements play a significant role in teaching and have value in their own right in giving the student information. Each of these is significant for later research. Further, it is generally acknowledged that teaching practical courses in the form of experiments has high learning value. The issue becomes more complex when animals are used as part of the experimental method and the students perform an "experiment" not to uncover new and potentially unknown information but to gain experience and confirm for themselves that which is already known. It can be argued that each of these objectives has high value but that the use of live animals demands a more rigid evaluation of the teaching objectives.

Many of the processes involved in biomedical research can be defined and expressed in terms of mathematical models. One of the goals of biomedical research is the expression of experimentally derived data in a statistically relevant form. Increasing in-depth investigation has given rise to information regarding biological phenomena that can be described mathematically. There is a historical development that has refined the depth of information from fairly simple global physiological data – cutting the vagus brings about a speeding up of the heart – to complex interrelated feedback models that involve hormonal, neurochemical and electric data. As a system is investigated, the level of information that becomes available increases, and sets of complex interrelationships will often develop. Mathematical expression of this data is called an algorithm. Computer science has allowed biomedical algorithms to be expressed with a high degree of accuracy. Computer presentation of data is usually in the form of text, graphics, and calculated graphic data (modelling). A good example of a complex simulation algorithm is that of the multifactorial control of blood glucose by insulin. A simulation model representing diabetes dynamics has been developed by Richmond (Figure 12-1; Richmond, 1990). This model is based on the integration of approximately 50 discrete physiological parameter "compartments." The combined simulation model is then manipulated to allow the study of changes in the parameters. The curve (Figure 12-1) represents four of the parameter subsystems.

In the past, computers presented graphic information (pictures, video, or animation) rather poorly. New generation computer systems have changed this situation with the result

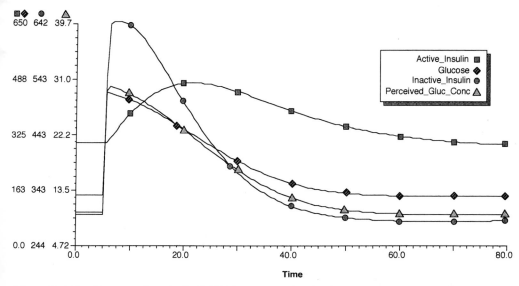

Figure 12-1. Graphic output from the Stella® Diabetes Dynamics simulation showing the concentration/time interrelationship between active insulin (■), glucose (◆), inactive insulin (●) and perceived glucose (▲) concentrations in the serum (Richmond, 1990).

that biomedical education software now consists of text, calculated data, and sophisticated graphics combined to give a high degree of realism. Software operating systems have also changed the way students interact with the computer. The human-machine interface has also changed so as to allow persons with little computer knowledge to use a computer with little, if any, previous training. All that is necessary is pointing and clicking with the help of a "mouse" (a cursor pointing device used to activate areas of the computer screen, allowing program instructions to be carried out). These developments have led to software designed to serve as true alternatives to animals in teaching.

Broadly speaking, computerized educational systems can be divided into three main classes of applications: a) pure software solutions that present data without making use of videotape or disk images; b) integrated courseware, which may make use of video; and c) virtual reality applications. Computer technology used as an educational tool has led to simulations, emulations, courseware, interactive video, computer controlled mannequins, and to virtual reality.

12.3 Software

Software applications that present biologically derived algorithms can be divided into two main categories: simulations and emulations.

Simulations present data that is both quantitatively and qualitatively correct. There are several types of applications that cover topics in physiology and pharmacology. Typical for these is that they allow manipulation of model parameters resulting in accurate presentations of data together with graphic presentation.

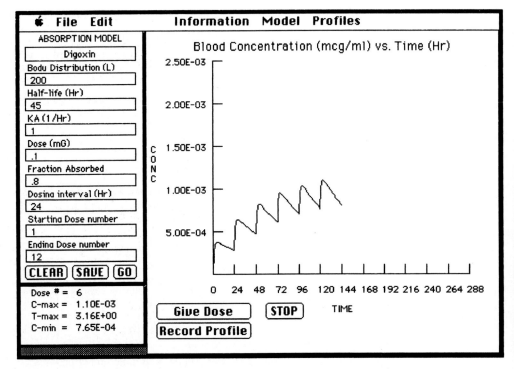

Figure 12-2. The PharMACokinetix® pharmacokinetic model of digitalis in a 30-kg dog. The curve shows the plasma concentration of the drug following 6 doses. The curve is calculated according to the kinetic model parameters shown to the left of the curve (Straugn and Rackley, 1990).

Pharmacokinetic programs can be designed to present drug plasma concentrations in terms of kinetic models. The model parameters can be designed to fit data derived from different species and in this way drug kinetics can be studied in several animal species (Figure 12-2; Straugn and Rackley, 1990).

There are distinct animal welfare benefits to be gained by using computer modelled pharmacokinetic simulations. The most apparent of these is that the computer allows students to administer drugs at toxic or even lethal levels without having to subject animals to potentially distressing procedures. The metabolism of many drugs spans several hours. In teaching student laboratory classes with animals, this would imply using several animals for each drug series or combination. Computer models allow repeated drug administration in various combinations and concentrations in the same "animal" and at much shorter time intervals (Blackman, 1983; Hughes, 1984b, 1988; Straugn and Rackley, 1990).

Physiology simulations have been designed to cover several commonly taught student practicals. There are several excellent applications available covering a wide range of phenomena, such as muscle physiology – including summation, tetanus, isometric contraction and the effects of curare depolarisation agents – or cardiac physiology and the effects of α- and β-adrenergic drugs on the heart. Similar applications exist for isolated ileum and gastric mucosa preparations (Hughes, 1984a), together with programs that display cardiac physiology (Figures 12-3a and 12-3b) (Peterson, 1989).

The second type of application makes use of a more graphic approach. *Emulation* software such as the PharmaTutor program (Keller, 1991) presents the physiological model with a high degree of realism but without the same degree of quantitative accuracy. The PharmaTutor experiment on the effects of acetylcholine on the heart shows representative blood pressure and heart rate readouts (Figure 12-4). These data are, however, not correct for the rat and must be seen more as a presentation of the principles embodied in the physiological or pharmacological experiments that the application is designed to model. On the other hand, the student gets a feel for the experimental setup and can study the principles embodied in the program in a pedagogically correct fashion (Keller, 1987). The PharmaTutor program also allows study without having to make use of accessory laser videodisk imagery.

12.4   Courseware

Many computer programs are limited to narrow descriptions of the biological phenomena they are designed to simulate. It is often necessary for the student to make use of accessory text books or manuals to get a more complete picture of the subject matter. There are also other areas of biomedical teaching that often make use of animals in other forms: handling, surgery, anesthesia, etc. The courseware concept embodies the presentation of teaching materials on the computer as an extended textbook or manual. Text and graphics in the form of either animated graphics or accessory video imagery are combined to allow the student to study a biomedical topic on the computer. The programs can be written in such a way as to allow the student to interact with the computer in an active two-way process instead of a passive one-way information flow from the source (textbook/manual) to the reader (student).

Our courseware package on the anesthesia and analgesia of laboratory animals has several sections that can be used as replacements and refinements of the use of live animals (Fosse and Hem, 1992; Nab, 1990b). These cover the handling of animals (intraperitoneal injection), the effects of atropine on the heart and gastrointestinal tract, and demonstrations of reflexes (cornea, pedal reflexes). This program is primarily designed to provide a one-way flow of information. The student uses the computer to access information and there is relatively little interaction with the program.

Interactivity is a characteristic of computer-aided teaching that makes this type of methodology particularly attractive when teaching courses that make use of animals. The rodent anesthesia programs designed by Nab (Nab, 1990a), and the interactive multimedia teaching programs on muscle physiology by Meijer (Meijer, 1992) are good examples of two-way teaching. These authors have prepared laser (video) disks that cover a wide range of scenarios that can be used as responses to questions or choices that the student must answer during the course of the program. Procedures involving animals are shown. Sequences cover the preparation of the experimental setup and the responses to various stimuli. The general design of such programs is based on the computer asking for a suitable answer and the student answering with a suitable response, either as textual reply or as a video playback of an appropriate sequence. The advantage of this type of interactive courseware is that it offers a high degree of realism with color video presentation of responses. The student can repeat sequences as often as necessary and can spend as much time as needed to gain the required level of information. It is necessary to use animals when preparing the video material but this occurs only once. The video disk can also be used by other authors. The Nab laser disk contains

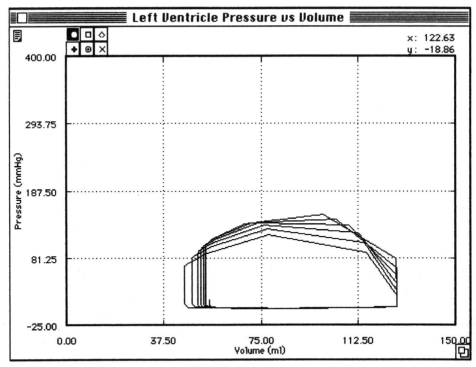

a

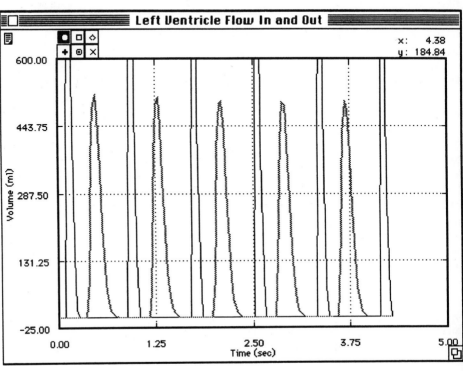

b

sequences that could be applied to the Fosse courseware on anesthesia (Fosse and Hem, 1992; Nab, 1990a). This in itself could lead to reductions in the numbers of animals needed to produce suitable video disks.

12.5   Interactive video

One of the commonest objections to the use of computerized alternatives to animals has been the fact that they do not give a true picture of the experimental setup coupled to hands-on experience with the biological preparation. In some respects this is correct. The advent of computer controlled video laser disks has, however, greatly expanded the degree of realism that can be obtained when teaching student practicals. Not only have film, slides, and video tape all been used in an attempt to enrich and enhance biomedical teaching, but they have also played a significant role in serving as alternatives to animals. However, they all suffer from significant drawbacks. Slides are static pictures that give no information about the relevant

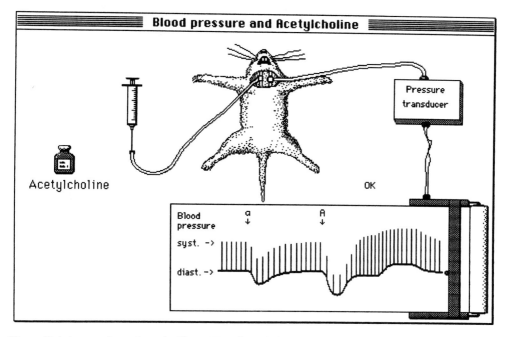

Figure 12-4. An experiment from the PharmaTutor® emulation (Keller, 1991). The experimental setup shows a rat with a catheter placed in the jugular for drug administration, and a pressure transducer catheter in the carotid artery. Blood pressure and heart rate is displayed following the administration of low and high doses of acetylcholine.

Figures 12-3a, 12-3b. Cardiac physiology models generated by a computer simulation system. Figure 12-3a shows the left ventricle pressure vs. volume curve. Figure 12-3b shows the left ventricle flow (in and out). The curves are generated by the Integrated Heart Laboratory software package (Peterson, 1989).

movement of the preparation in the experimental setup. Film presents the information in a linear fashion that is determined at the time of production. This makes it difficult to access sequences placed in the middle of a film which may be needed as a part of a teaching program. This would entail winding the film to the sequence, showing it, and then returning to the previous location. The same problem is encountered when using video tape as a medium for interactive teaching. The key to interactivity is the ability to present several scenarios and options to the student. This allows the student to reply to questions, or to choose pathways in an attempt to solve problems that the experiment poses. The advent of computer controlled video (laser) disks or CD-ROM discs provided the degree of rapid pathway selection needed for interactive teaching.

Video disks allow storage of vast amounts of pictorial and sound material. Sequences representing several possible scenarios to a problem can be recorded on the disk and computer software written to allow playback irrespective of the order of recording. This has clear implications when designing teaching programs. In contrast to film or video tape, which must be wound either forwards or backwards when accessing non-sequential scenes, the disk allows the student to play back sequences almost instantaneously. Laser disks require special playback equipment. The disk can be either played back on a separate television monitor, or overlaid on the computer screen. In other teaching systems, bar codes can be generated and printed in student manuals (Figure 12-5). The student reads the bar code by means of a barcode pen and the computer controller plays the sequence on the disk. The Norwegian Veterinary College has developed student manuals using this type of approach. The Ciba Geigy video disk on pharmacologic and toxicologic responses to drugs is used to illustrate principles of anesthesia, pharmacology, and toxicology (A. Smith, personal communication).

A significant disadvantage of the use of laser disks is the cost of producing and recording the master disk and its subsequent pressing. This is a process that requires expert help and is not something that an average teacher can undertake. There are, however, several disks that have been produced by commercial and other university sources. These disks cover a series of topics ranging from the pharmacological and toxicological effects of drugs to cardiac and muscle physiology and the anesthesia of small rodents. Provided they are given the directory of the material on the disk, users will be able to write their own programs and include the material on the disk. There is a vast potential for this medium, and the advent of new optical storage disks will make the process of making new video disks simpler and more accessible for average users.

12.6   Computer controlled mannequins

Models have been used for teaching purposes for many years. The first models were wax representations of internal organs and were used for teaching anatomy and pathology. The advent of modern plastic materials allowed the production of models that were no longer mere static copies. These models allowed biomedical students to practice procedures such as intubation, laparoscopy, and other procedures that otherwise would have had to be performed on either human or animal subjects. A major breakthrough occurred when computer technology was coupled to plastic models. Instead of having a static dummy as a subject, the computer was used to simulate organ responses to manipulation. Models have been made that allow the training of cardiac arrest reversal. Here a plastic torso is coupled to electrocardio-

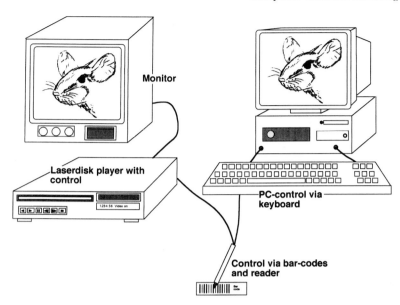

Figure 12-5. Interactive video by means of laser disk. Video images and sequences on the disk can be played directly on a television monitor, controlled by computers and integrated within courseware or controlled by bar codes embedded in text. (Reproduced with the permission of R.T. Fosse from *Animals in Biomedical Research*. Edited by J. Hau and P. Svendsen. CRC Press, NY, in press.)

graph recorders and the chest is motorized so as to "breathe" realistically. The heart can be auscultated with a stethoscope and the patient can be intubated. A series of cardiac emergencies can be simulated, and the computer controls the responses of the model to the manipulations or treatments that are performed. Similar models have been produced for use in automobile crash testing. The General Motors Corporation BIOSID model was developed using data derived from animal-based testing. The BIOSID model and a similar General Motors computer-driven model HYBRID III have to a large extent replaced the use of dogs and pigs in crash testing (K.L. Smiler, personal communication).

12.7   Virtual reality

All human sensory and motor response is based on input of sensory information together with the ability to spatially associate the sensory input within space and time. Sound and images have been available in forms that readily allow computerization. Examples of this are discussed in the section on laser disk technology. The idea behind virtual reality is based on an integration of these elements in forms that give the user an impression of participation. This can best be described by looking at the way pictures are presented on computers. In a conventional display system, this is done by means of a screen that displays a television-like image to the viewer. Similarly, sound is presented via loudspeakers and may be stereo or monaural.

New technology has brought about totally different concepts in image presentation. The aerospace industry has long had so-called head up displays, in which instruments are displayed on semitransparent glass screens that allow aircraft pilots to read instruments without looking down, thus maintaining the surrounding field of view. This has led to specially designed helmets that allow a viewer to see the computer image within a floating field of vision. This gives the impression of being inside the image. At the same time, sound is presented through a stereo headset. The illusion is developed further by wearing gloves with sensors that analyze the positioning of the hands and fingers and translate this into spatial information that can be analyzed and used in controlling the image in the helmet. Images are recorded on laser disks capable of storing the vast number of sequences needed, and computer software controls the integration of imagery with sound and spatial information derived from gloves or other body mounted sensors (Pimentel and Texeira, 1993; Sherhouse *et al.*, 1990; Sherhouse and Chaney, 1991; Woolley, 1992).

Several models have been proposed for virtual reality imagery. The most likely of these is the development of surgery training systems in which three-dimensional anatomy images are controlled by the computer. The user holds surgical instruments and "operates" on the computer image. The spatial sensory information that comes from the gloves is used to relate the position of the instrument to the computerized image. This would allow the surgeon to cut though blood vessels which would bleed or through other structures which would then respond accordingly. The computer can be programmed to interact with the surgeon and give information as errors are made (Sherhouse *et al.*, 1990; Sherhouse and Chaney, 1991).

The technology is still at a very early stage of development but will probably develop rapidly as computing power increases and image storage improves. There is considerable promise for this type of technology as a replacement for animals used for surgery training or anatomical dissection.

12.8   Conclusion

Computer assisted teaching in biomedical education is a new and rapidly developing method. Despite resistance from teachers who are used to teaching with animals, this process should be encouraged and developed. Several databases have been developed that list available software that can be used as alternatives to animals in education (Bernatzky *et al.*, 1992; Smith *et al.*, 1993). New developments in computer and software technology will greatly enhance the quality of teaching programs. There will be an ever increasing degree of reality. There are clear pedagogic advantages to teaching in this way. It is also clear that it is possible to replace many of the animals that are used to teach well-known and established theory.

References

Bernatzky G., Renz S. and Scheuber P. H. (1992) *Wissen schützt Tiere. Ein Katalog über Ergänzungs- und Ersatzmethoden zum Tierversuch in Ausbildung und Lehre.* Naturwissenschaftliche Fakultät der Universität Salzburg, Salzburg.

Blackman J. G. (1983) Microcomputer simulation of pharmacokinetic behaviour of drugs for teaching and learning. *British Journal of Pharmacology* **80**(Suppl.), 589.

Fosse R. T. and Hem A. (1992) *Anesthesia and Analgesia of Laboratory Animals* [Computer program]. NIF Software, Norwegian Resource Group for Laboratory Animal Science, Oslo.

Hughes I. (1984a) *Ileum* [Computer program]. Elseviers Biosoft, Cambridge.

Hughes I. E. (1984b) The use of computers to simulate animal preparations in the teaching of practical pharmacology. *ATLA* **11**, 204–213.

Hughes I. E. (1988) A computer simulated anterior tibialis-sciatic nerve preparation (in-vivo) for teaching neuromuscular pharmacology. *British Journal of Pharmacology* **93**(Suppl.), 307.

Keller D. (1987) Pharmakologie-Unterricht am Computer. *ALTEX* **Nr. 7**, 5–11.

Keller D. (1991) *PharmaTutor* [Computer program]. Fonds für versuchstierfreie Forschung, Zürich.

Meijer N. W. (1992) *Muscle Physiology* [Computer program]. Department of Physiology, University of Groningen, Groningen.

Nab J. (1990a) *Anesthesia in the Rat* [Computer program]. Department of Laboratory Animal Science, Utrecht University, Utrecht.

Nab J. (1990b). Reduction of animal experiments in education in the Netherlands. *ATLA* **18**, 57–63.

Peterson N. (1989) *Integrated Heart Laboratory* [Computer program]. Command Applied Technology, Monmouth, Oregon.

Pimentel K. and Texeira K. (1993) *Virtual Reality – Through the New Looking Glass.* Intel/Windcrest/McGraw Hill Inc., New York.

Richmond B. (1990) *Diabetes Dynamics Using STELLA®* [Computer program]. High Performance Systems, Hannover, NH.

Sherhouse G. W., Bourland J. D., Reynolds K., McMurry H. L., Mitchell T. P. and Chaney E. L. (1990) Virtual simulation in the clinical setting: some practical considerations. *International Journal of Radiation and Oncological Biology and Physiology* **19**, 1059–1065.

Sherhouse G. W. and Chaney E. L. (1991) The portable virtual simulator. *International Journal of Radiation and Oncological Biology and Physiology* **21**, 475–483.

Smith A., Smith I. and Fosse R. T. (1993) *NORINA: Norwegian Inventory of Audiovisuals – A Database on Audiovisual and Computer Based Training Methods.* Norwegian College of Veterinary Medicine, Oslo.

Straugn A. and Rackley R. (1990) *PharMACokinetix* [Computer program]. University of Tennessee, Memphis.

Woolley B. (1992) *Virtual Worlds.* Blackwell Publishers, Oxford.

13 Alternatives to Experiments with Animals in Medical Education: A TEMPUS Joint European Project

Miroslav Červinka, Zuzana Červinková, Michael Balls, and Horst Spielmann

Summary

The Trans-European Mobility Scheme for University Studies (TEMPUS Program) was adopted by the Council of Ministers of the European Communities in 1990 to support the reform process in Eastern Europe in the field of higher education. Central to the TEMPUS Program is the development of Joint European Projects (JEPs) based on the participation of universities from East European countries and partner organizations in EC Member States. One JEP involves cooperation among the University of Nottingham, the Free University of Berlin, FRAME (Nottingham), ZEBET (Berlin) and the Charles University Medical Faculty in Hradec Králové. The main goal of this JEP is to introduce the Three Rs concept and practical approaches to alternatives to animal experiments into the educational system of the universities of the Czech Republic and so to promote their development in Eastern Europe.

Abbreviations. FRAME = Fund for the Replacement of Animals in Medical Experiments; JEP = Joint European Project; TEMPUS = Trans-European Mobility Scheme for University Studies; ZEBET = Zentralstelle zur Erfassung und Bewertung von Ergänzungs- und Ersatzmethoden zum Tierversuch (Center for Documentation and Evaluation of Alternative Methods to Animal Experiments).

13.1 The rationale and background of the project

Every year, millions of laboratory animals are used in biomedical experiments in research and education. Recently, there has been a strong movement in most industrialized countries toward finding alternatives to these animal experiments. The term *alternative* has a special meaning in this context, as it is used to embrace all the Three Rs of Russell and Burch (1959) namely, the Reduction, Refinement and Replacement of animal procedures. The rationale for this effort is based on scientific, economic and ethical considerations. Reform on the basis of the Three Rs is required in the Member States of the EC under the terms of Directive 86/609/EEC in all fields, including higher education, as well as research and testing. Therefore we appreciate the establishment of the TEMPUS program.

Alternatives to Animal Testing. New Ways in the Biomedical Sciences, Trends and Progress.
Reinhardt, C.A. (ed.). 1994. © VCH, Weinheim.

The TEMPUS Program (the acronym for Trans-European Mobility Scheme for University Studies) was adopted by the Council of Ministers of the European Communities in 1990 to support the reform process in Eastern Europe in the field of higher education. At the center of the TEMPUS Program is the development of Joint European Projects (JEPs) based on the participation of universities from East European countries and partner organizations in EC Member States.

The JEP described here arises from long-established contacts between the Charles University Medical Faculty in Hradec Králové (Department of Biology) and the Nottingham University Medical School (Department of Human Morphology). The detailed outline of the JEP was discussed during a short visit (sponsored by a TEMPUS Mobility Grant) by M. Červinka to Nottingham in February 1991. There are five participating organizations included in this project:

- The University of Nottingham, Department of Human Morphology; contact person: M. Balls;
- FRAME (Fund for the Replacement of Animals in Medical Experiments); contact person: M. Balls, Chairman of the Trustees;
- The Free University of Berlin; contact person: H. Spielmann;
- ZEBET (Zentralstelle zur Erfassung und Bewertung von Ergänzungs- und Ersatzmethoden zum Tierversuch), established in 1989 by the Bundesgesundheitsamt (Federal Health Office) in Berlin; contact person: H. Spielmann, Director;
- The Medical Faculty of Charles University, Hradec Králové; contact person: M. Červinka, Coordinator of the JEP.

The main goal of this JEP is to introduce both the Three Rs concept and practical approaches to alternatives to animal experiments in the universities of the Czech Republic and so to enhance their scientific, economic, and social relevance. Furthermore, this will lead to an enhancement of the quality of education within the Czech Republic through the theoretical and practical retraining of teachers, bringing them fully up to date with the latest state-of-the-art information in this fast-moving field.

13.2   Planned cooperation activities

The cooperation activities planned comprise a series of coordinated training visits by university teachers from Hradec Králové to Nottingham and Berlin. This will be complemented by short training/advisory visits by experienced university staff from Nottingham and Berlin to Hradec Králové. The targets to be met are the:

- training of the Hradec Králové University teaching staff in modern in vitro techniques and their incorporation into practical classes;
- development of teaching packages on alternative methodology for students;
- facilitation of interaction at the staff and student levels among the participating institutions;
- preparation of procedural recommendations for the use of animals for educational purposes in medical faculties;
- preparation of a final report (as a basis for discussion at the final evaluation meeting).

The overall result should be significant improvements in:

- the curricula of the medical faculties (e. g. lectures about the concept of alternatives and the ethics of animal experimentation);
- the work of ethical committees in medical faculties;
- the preparation of new rules and regulations for controlling the use of animals in education and research in medical faculties;
- training in the practical use of alternative methods;
- the production and exchange of the new teaching materials concerning alternatives;
- discussions among staff and students about the scientific and ethical value of alternative approaches.

The project should provide strategies that will be of value both to other faculties in higher education and to institutional ethical committees elsewhere in the Czech Republic and in other Eastern European countries.

The training envisaged will involve training visits of four months in total per year by three to four members of the Charles University Medical Faculty teaching staff (from the Departments of Biology, Physiology, Pharmacology, and Surgery) to Nottingham and to Berlin. Each visit will allow two to three weeks for observing the operation of the curriculum, attending relevant practical classes and lectures, collecting information about alternatives, discussing the use of the alternatives in education and research, collecting educational material, and participating in the work of alternatives laboratories. The training visits will be interspersed with, and complemented by, a series of short training/consultation visits (two to three weeks) by coordinating staff from Nottingham and Berlin to Hradec Králové.

In the first year (1991–1992), the main activity was a detailed comparison of the curriculum of the Medical Faculty of Charles University with that of Nottingham University Medical School, with special emphasis on how the practical classes using animals in Hradec Králové could be replaced. A similar comparison with teaching practices in Berlin then followed. The second main activity involved training in the concept of alternatives and in the development and validation of alternative methods, especially replacement, for use in education, research, and testing. This comprised a coordinated program, so that the experience gained in Nottingham and Berlin was complementary, not duplicative.

Emphasis in the second year (1992–1993) will be on particular parts of medical education (e. g. computer program development, toxicokinetics) and particular safety problems (e. g. ocular and dermal irritancy, teratogenicity, carcinogenicity, immunotoxicity, neurotoxicity), including the production of interactive video programs and protocols for practical classes involving in vitro techniques. The role of information resources, including literature-based and technique-based databases, will also be covered.

Emphasis in the third year (1993–1994) will be on agreements and proposals for curriculum review, including the introduction of courses on biomedical ethics and practical classes involving non-animal methods, both as replacements for animal procedures and as methods of choice for use in biomedical education, research, and teaching. In addition, active steps will be taken to set up discussions with other medical faculties in the Czech Republic, and with other institutions, not only in the U. K. and Germany, but also in other EC Member States (e. g. through the European Research Group for Alternatives in Toxicity Testing (ERGATT), of which M. Balls and H. Spielmann are members) and in other Eastern European countries.

There will be a final evaluation meeting in Hradec Králové upon completion of this project, bringing together representatives from all the partner organizations. They will prepare a final report, including recommendations for curriculum development, ethical committee guidelines, etc., suitable for all medical faculties in the Czech Republic and elsewhere.

13.3   Overview of activities 1991–1992

The first steps were taken in the fall of 1991. The participants of the JEP in Hradec Králové started to collect information about the actual use of animals in medical education in the Czech Republic. Information on the use of laboratory animals in education in the departments of the university (species, purpose, and number of animals per year) is now available.

In order to update knowledge in the field of alternatives, it was necessary to supply the participants in Hradec Králové with recent information on this subject. Therefore the participants from EC countries started sending the coordinator of the JEP the issues of *ATLA* (*Alternatives to Laboratory Animals*) on a regular basis, as well as information concerning the INVITTOX database. The coordinator also received new material about ZEBET – the National German Center for Alternatives to Animal Experiments at the Federal Health Office in Berlin – and information about the ZEBET alternatives databank.

Further, the grant provided the Department of Biology in Hradec Králové with essential equipment for carrying out the proposed program, namely a personal computer, which will be used for handling laboratory data and storing information about alternatives, CO_2 tissue culture incubators, a laminar flow sterile bench, and a microplate reader. This equipment is necessary for in vitro cell culture.

The most important activities involve personal contacts among the participants. During the first year of the JEP, two participants from Charles University visited the medical faculty in Nottingham and FRAME. During these visits, the curricula of both medical faculties were compared. One of the visitors received practical laboratory training in cell culture work. Two teachers from the medical faculty in Hradec Králové visited ZEBET and the Free University in Berlin, also with the aim of comparing the curricula of the two medical faculties.

In return, M. Balls, R. Clothier (Nottingham), and H. Spielmann visited the medical faculty in Hradec Králové on the occasion of a symposium, during which the academic staff and students were thoroughly informed about the situation in the European Community, and the situation in the Czech Republic was discussed. About 50 people attended the symposium, some of them from other universities in the Czech Republic. This symposium was effective in changing opinion among both students and teachers.

There are already some positive results at the level of the medical faculty in Hradec Králové, even after only one year of participation in this project. The Scientific Board of the faculty discussed the question of the use of animals in the faculty and officially concluded that the main task of the current academic year should be the preparation of special rules for the use of laboratory animals in education and research in the faculty. Another important step was taken at the level of the departments. The curricula are now being revised, and most of the teachers are trying to reduce the use of laboratory animals. We hope that the experience of this faculty can be transferred in the near future to other medical faculties in the Czech Republic.

Acknowledgement. We thank the Commission of the European Communities for support of this project (JEP-1485–91–1).

Reference

Russell W. M. S. and Burch R. L. (1959) *The Principles of Humane Experimental Technique.* Methuen & Co Ltd., London.

14 Replacement of Laboratory Animals in the Management of Blood-Sucking Arthropods

Achim E. Issmer, Thomas H. Schilling, Andreas Vollmer, and Jörg Grunewald

Summary

Blood-sucking arthropods transmit a variety of infectious agents. For the research on vector-borne diseases the maintenance of such vectors in the laboratory is inevitable. The feeding of these arthropods requires the blood of living animals, and the replacement of these laboratory animals used for blood-feeding is our primary objective. Artificial feeding techniques of different Diptera, e. g. *Aedes aegypti*, *Culicoides nubeculosus* and Simuliidae, or bugs, such as *Triatoma infestans*, *Dipetalogaster maximus* and *Rhodnius prolixus*, and of the soft tick *Ornithodorus moubata* have been established in our laboratory. Most recently, we also developed an artificial membrane feeding technique for the adults of the hard ticks *Hyalomma truncatum* and *Ixodes ricinus*, as well as for the blood-feeding stages of the mite *Ornithonyssus bacoti*.

14.1 Introduction

Haematophagous arthropods carry and transmit a variety of pathogenic and parasitic organisms to man and animals, causing debilitating diseases and the loss of billions of dollars in agriculture. Major human vector-borne diseases include malaria, filariasis, trypanosomiasis, leishmaniasis, yellow fever, dengue fever, Lyme disease, and encephalitis as well as other virus and bacterial diseases.

The development of suitable methods for therapy and the control of cyclically transmitted parasitoses requires knowledge of the epidemiology and the biology of the causative organisms, their hosts, and their vectors. Regular blood meals are indispensable for the maintenance of these arthropods as well as for their infestation with the respective parasite. This has required the use of laboratory animals for blood-feeding. Alternative methods which partially or completely replace the laboratory animal save animal lives, expenses, and ideally allow the maintenance of the parasite-host cycle in vitro. For several years our laboratory has maintained different filarial parasites, their hosts, and the respective vectors. The main emphasis of our research is the investigation of human onchocerciasis, a filarial infection with a wide distribution in Africa and also in parts of Latin America. The causative organism of this disease is the parasitic nematode *Onchocerca volvulus* (Filarioidea), which is trans-

Alternatives to Animal Testing. New Ways in the Biomedical Sciences, Trends and Progress.
Reinhardt, C. A. (ed.). 1994. © VCH, Weinheim.

mitted by several species of blackflies (Diptera: Simuliidae). Onchocerciasis (river blindness) is one of the major tropical diseases targeted for control by the World Health Organization.

Because *O. volvulus* is human specific, animal models have to be used alternatively for research on this filariasis. In our laboratory we have successfully established the complete life cycles of three filarial parasites:

- *Acanthocheilonema viteae* in the jird *Meriones unguiculatus* with the vector tick *Ornithodorus moubata* (Acari: Argasidae);
- *Litomosoides carinii* in the cotton rat *Sigmodon hispidus*, which is transmitted by the mite *Ornithonyssus bacoti* (Acari);
- *Monanema martini* in the African striped mouse *Lemniscomys striatus* and vector tick *Hyalomma truncatum* (Acari: Ixodidae).

Our primary objective is to drastically reduce the numbers of laboratory animals used in the maintenance of these filarial cycles, particularly during the breeding of the arthropod vectors.

In addition to the vectors in the life cycles of the filarial parasites, colonies of other vectors are also maintained:

- the hard tick *Ixodes ricinus* (Acari: Ixodidae), vector of several bacteria (e. g. *Borrelia burgdorferi*; Lyme disease) and viruses (encephalitis):
- bugs (*Triatoma infestans*, *Rhodnius prolixus* and *Dipetalogaster maximus* (Hemiptera: Reduviidae)) which transmit *Trypanosoma cruzi* (Chagas disease in South America);
- the mosquito *Aedes aegypti* (Diptera: Culicidae), the vector of the yellow fever and dengue fever viruses and of *Dirofilaria immitis* (heart worm disease);
- biting midges, *Culicoides nubeculosus* (Diptera: Ceratopogonidae), the vector of *Onchocerca gutturosa*, a parasitic filaria of cattle;
- several species of Simuliidae (Diptera) which transmit *Onchocerca lienalis* and *O. tarsicola*, parasitic filariae of cattle and red deer.

Based on our experience with the artificial membrane-feeding of Diptera and soft ticks, we have further developed these feeding techniques for hard ticks and mites. These methods were adapted to the different blood-feeding behaviour of the various arthropods, i. e. different blood sources (sheep, cattle, pig, etc.), temperature, membrane types, and supplements.

However, alternative methods have to guarantee the same quality and quantity of parasitic material, which is needed for the ongoing biomedical research and also for teaching activities.

A control measure of the quality of an artificial membrane-feeding technique is the fecundity of the blood-fed arthropod, compared with that of those fed in vivo. These alternative membrane-feeding systems are successfully used as a substitute for in vivo feeding for the breeding of *Ae. aegypti*, *C. nubeculosus*, *O. moubata* and partially for the Reduviidae. For the mite *O. bacoti*, a new technique and a new membrane for in vitro feeding has been developed. For adult hard ticks, artificial membrane feeding to repletion and successful oviposition was first described by Waladde *et al.* (1991). We have developed an artificial membrane and a new technique to feed the adults of *I. ricinus* and *H. truncatum* to repletion and to achieve successful oviposition.

14.2 Maintenance of the arthropods

14.2.1 Soft ticks (Argasidae)

The soft tick *O. moubata* is kept at 28 °C, a relative humidity of 80 ± 5 % and fed artificially, as described by Wirtz and Barthold (1986). With this technique, laboratory animals as a blood source are no longer required. Rodents are kept only for the maintenance of filariae in their natural host, and approaches to further reduce the number of animals required are currently being investigated (Rapp *et al.*, 1994, this volume).

14.2.2 Hard ticks (Ixodidae)

The hard tick *H. truncatum* is kept in closed plastic vessels at 27 °C and 95 ± 2 % relative humidity. Hard ticks have one larval, one nymph, and one adult stage, and each stage has to take a blood meal which usually lasts several days. The larvae and the nymphs are fed on mice, the adult stage on rabbits. However, recently an artificial membrane-feeding technique for the adults of *H. truncatum* has been developed. This technique is also suitable for the adults of *I. ricinus*, collected in the field.

Although it was not possible to maintain a colony of hard ticks without a blood meal on animals, artificial feeding of hard ticks is feasible. Possibilities of replacing the in vivo feeding of adult ticks are currently being investigated (A. E. Issmer, unpublished results). This would reduce the number of animals required for the filarial life cycle of *M. martini* and its vector tick *H. truncatum*.

14.2.3 Mites (Acari)

The mite *O. bacoti* is kept in a separate room in glass boxes filled with timber chips. The boxes are placed in a basin filled with glycerol to prevent this arthropod from escaping. The room temperature is adjusted to 25 °C, the relative humidity to 90 ± 5 %. Previously, the mites were regularly blood-fed on a rodent which was placed inside the box for about 4 hr. Currently, a device for the artificial feeding of the mites is used, which is a modified technique previously described by Wenk and Lantow (1982) (T. H. Schilling, unpublished results). The maintenance of mites without animals as a blood source has been carried on for more than three generations.

14.2.4 Bugs (Reduviidae)

The bugs *Rhodnius prolixus*, *Dipetalogaster maximus* and *Triatoma infestans* are kept in small plastic containers in a room at 80 ± 5 % relative humidity and 28 °C. For blood-feeding, an anaesthetized white mouse or rat is placed into the rearing containers. An artificial membrane feeding technique is currently being evaluated, and the effects of different blood sources (sheep, man, etc.) and membranes (Parafilm M™, American National Can) on the fecundity of the female bugs are also being investigated (Figure 14-1).

Although in triatomine bugs artificial membrane feeding techniques are used by several laboratories, a reduced fertility and an increased mortality has been observed (Gardiner and Maddrell, 1972). In order to maintain a permanent colony and a constant number of vectors, the bugs still have to be fed from time to time on anesthetized mice and rats. In our laboratory promising progress has been made toward completely replacing the animal by membrane-feeding. (A. Vollmer, unpublished results).

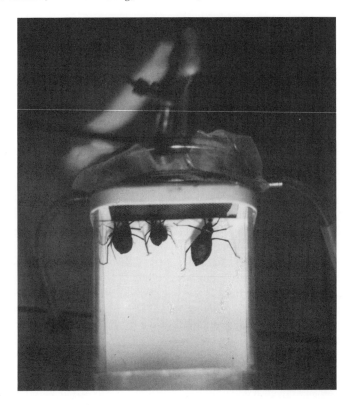

Figure 14-1. Artificial feeding of *Dipetalogaster maximus* UHLER 1894 (Hemiptera: Reduviidae). Four larvae (left) and one adult female (right) are sucking the sheep blood (50 units heparin/ml). The feeding apparatus is made of aluminum and the water heated (37 °C); the membrane is Parafilm M™.

14.2.5   Diptera

The mosquito *Ae. aegypti* has been maintained in our laboratory for several years and reared according to the method of Hagen and Grunewald (1990).

Also various blackfly species (Simuliidae) were collected in the field and reared and blood-fed according to the techniques described by Grunewald (1973), Raybould and Grunewald (1975), Grunewald and Wirtz (1978), and Rutschke and Grunewald (1984).

The pre-imaginal stages and the adults of the biting midge *C. nubeculosus* (Diptera: Ceratopogonidae) are reared according to techniques that were developed in our laboratory (Fahrner and Barthelmess, 1988; Fahrner *et al.*, 1988). The females are fed on cattle blood through latex membranes using a feeding apparatus originally developed for the feeding of Simuliidae (Grunewald and Wirtz, 1978; Wirtz, 1985).

The breeding of *Ae. aegypti*, *C. nubeculosus* and the Simuliidae requires no animals. The artificial feeding on membranes is well established, easy to handle, and cheaper than the use of animals.

14.3   Conclusion

In our laboratory several techniques for the artificial blood-feeding of arthropod vectors have been developed and successfully applied to replace laboratory animals as a blood source. For the breeding and maintenance of soft ticks no animals are required. Also vectors such as *Ae. aegypti* and *C. nubeculosus* and some triatomine bugs can be maintained in the laboratory without the use of living animals as blood donors.

For the maintenance of mite and hard tick colonies new membrane feeding techniques have recently been established. This will drastically reduce the number of mammals as blood donors as well. However, laboratory animals will still be needed to maintain rodent filariae life cycles as models for human pathogenic filariases. Nevertheless, for some developmental stages of filarial parasites the in vitro cultivation could offer a possibility for replacing mammals as experimental hosts (Rapp *et al.*, 1994, this volume). Further studies are required to reduce the use of small mammals for the maintenance of filarial life cycles in the laboratory.

References

Fahrner J. and Barthelmess C. (1988) Rearing of *Culicoides nubeculosus* (Diptera: Ceratopogonidae) by natural or artificial feeding in the laboratory. *Veterinary Parasitology* **28**, 307–313.

Fahrner J., Vankan D. and Schulz-Key H. (1988) Ingestion of microfilariae from different sources by *Culicoides nubeculosus* (Diptera: Ceratopogonidae) through an artificial membrane. *Veterinary Parasitology* **28**, 315–320.

Gardiner B. O. C. and Maddrell S. H. P. (1972) Techniques for routine and large-scale rearing of *Rhodnius prolixus* Stål (Hem., Reduviidae). *Bulletin of Entomological Research* **61**, 505–515.

Grunewald J. (1973) Die hydrochemischen Lebensbedingungen der präimaginalen Stadien von *Boophtera erythrocephala* De Geer (Diptera, Simuliidae). 2. Die Entwicklung einer Zucht unter experimentellen Bedingungen. *Zeitschrift für Tropenmedizin und Parasitologie* **24**, 232–249.

Grunewald J. and Wirtz H. P. (1978) Künstliche Blutfütterung einiger afrikanischer und palaearktischer Simuliiden (Diptera). *Zeitschrift für angewandte Entomologie* **85**, 425–435.

Hagen H. E. and Grunewald J. (1990) Routine blood-feeding of *Aedes aegypti* via a new membrane. *Journal of the American Mosquito Association* **6**, 535–536.

Rapp J., Hoffmann W. H., Keller L., Welzel A. and Schulz-Key, H. (1994) Maintenance of filarial cycles in the laboratory: Approaches to replacing the vertebrate host. In *Alternatives to Animal Testing. New Ways in the Biomedical Sciences, Trends and Progress*. Edited by C. A. Reinhardt. pp. 131–139. VCH Verlagsgesellschaft, Weinheim.

Raybould J. N. and Grunewald J. (1975) Present progress towards the laboratory colonization of African Simuliidae (Diptera). *Tropenmedizin und Parasitologie* **26**, 155–168.

Rutschke J. and Grunewald J. (1984) A simple apparatus for maintaining black fly adults (Simuliidae) in the laboratory. *Mosquito News* **44**, 461–465.

Waladde S. M., Ochieng S. A. and Gichuhi P. M. (1991) Artificial-membrane feeding of the ixodid tick *Rhipicephalus appendiculatus*, to repletion. *Experimental and Applied Acarology* **11**, 297–306.

Wenk P. and Lantow S. (1982) Infestation der Milbe *Ornithonyssus bacoti* Hirt 1913 (Acari) mit Microfilarien von *Litomosoides carinii* Chandler 1931 (Nematoda, Filarioidea) bei künstlicher Fütterung mit Blut von Baumwollratten *Sigmodon hispidus*. *Zeitschrift für angewandte Entomologie* **93**, 523–532.

Wirtz H. P. (1985) Nahrungsaufnahme und Natalitaet bei palaearktischen Simuliiden (Diptera). 2. Blutfütterung von *Boophtera erythrocephala* De Geer, 1776 und *Wilhelmia lineata*, Meigen, 1804, durch Membranen. *Zeitschrift für angewandte Entomologie* **99**, 377–393.

Wirtz H. P. and Barthold E. (1986) Simplified membrane feeding of *Ornithodorus moubata* (Acarina: Argasidae) and quantitative transmission of microfilariae of *Dipetalonema viteae* (Nematoda: Filarioidea) to the ticks. *Zeitschrift für Angewandte Zoologie* **73**, 1–11.

15　Maintenance of Filarial Cycles in the Laboratory: Approaches to Replacing the Vertebrate Host

Joachim Rapp, Wolfgang H. Hoffmann, Lisette Keller, Andrea Welzel, and Hartwig Schulz-Key

Summary

Filarial infections are of great medical and social importance for people living in developing countries. Owing to the host specificity of human filariae, animal models from allied species are used to study the parasite host interaction or when developing new drugs. The maintenance of filarial cycles in the laboratory is still based on the infection of a considerable number of rodents. Alternative techniques permitting the gradual replacement of vertebrate hosts are presented here. These involve the artificial feeding of vectors and their infestation with microfilariae at membrane sites, followed by the cryopreservation of viable parasitic material for purposes of storage. While in vitro cultivation of filarial worms allows a rather limited replacement of vertebrate hosts, it is of high relevance for biochemical, immunological, and pharmacological studies. It is expected that the systematic development and application of these novel alternative techniques will significantly reduce (by more than 50 %) the number of rodents presently still required for filarial research.

15.1　Introduction

Over 100 million people in the tropics are infected by the parasitic nematodes *Wuchereria bancrofti*, *Brugia malayi*, or *Onchocerca volvulus*. These infections cause elephantiasis (lymphatic filariasis) or river blindness (onchocerciasis), which are of great medical, social and economic significance for poor populations of developing countries. Although vector control and mass chemotherapy have been successfully applied in some endemic areas, more effective drugs or a vaccine against these filarial parasites are urgently needed (World Health Organization, 1988). Hence the need to induce filarial infections in small animals for drug screening, immunological investigations, and vaccine tests.

　　Since human filariae are host specific, allied filarial species in rodents have been introduced in order to investigate the parasite-host interaction. Owing to the diverse parasitological, immunological, and pathological features of the human filariases, there is a need for a wide variety of models if the whole spectrum of clinical manifestations is to be reflected. Though in vitro techniques are of considerable value in special biochemical, immunological, or molecular biological investigations, they have proved to be inadequate in maintaining the

Alternatives to Animal Testing. New Ways in the Biomedical Sciences, Trends and Progress.
Reinhardt, C. A. (ed.). 1994. © VCH, Weinheim.

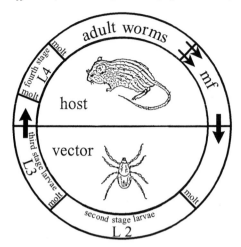

Figure 15-1. Scheme of the cycles of rodent filariae (*A. viteae, L. carinii, M. martini*). The outer cycle shows the different parasite stages and the parasitic infection phases. mf = microfilariae, L2–L4 = larval stages.

parasitic cycle outside the vertebrate or invertebrate host. Moreover, for most investigations of the parasite-host interaction the vertebrate cannot be replaced at all.

Maintenance of filarial cycles in the laboratory is rather laborious. Since the rodent filarial species are dependent on transmission by ticks or mites, colonies of these vectors have to be reared in order to produce sufficient infective larvae of the parasite (L3, Figure 15-1). Additionally, inbred strains are needed for immunological studies, and most experiments require well-defined parasitological or immunological properties in the vertebrate host. Finally, filarial cycles also need to be sustained in periods of low experimental activity. The vast majority of infected animals are used to maintain the delicate parasite-vector-host system or else are kept ready so that adequate viable parasitic material can be supplied as required. In other words, only a minor portion of infected animals are actually used in immunological or chemotherapeutical experiments. The total number of animals needed for filarial research could be significantly reduced if available alternative techniques were more reliable and efficient. We employ three proved approaches in our laboratory to replace or spare infected and uninfected animals:

- Cryopreservation of filarial stages isolated from the vertebrate host or the vector (microfilariae, infective stages). Thawed parasites can be used for maintenance of the cycle in the laboratory or for other purposes (Fahrner and Barthelmess, 1987; Fahrner et al., 1987). Cryopreservation of different stages of the arthropod vectors is envisaged as a further approach.
- Feeding and infestation of the vectors via artificial membranes, or via intra-thoracic or intra-abdominal injection of microfilariae into the vectors, in order to harvest infective larvae.
- In vitro cultivation of the different stages of the parasite in order to promote their further development.

We presently maintain in our laboratory three filarial cycles with different parasitological and immunological features. These are natural parasite-host systems. Adult worms of *Acanthocheilonema viteae* are located in subcutaneous tissues or in deeper layers between muscle fibers of *Meriones unguiculatus*. Their blood-dwelling microfilariae are characteristically unsheathed. They are taken up concomitantly with the blood meal by the soft tick *Ornithodoros moubata,* in which they then develop to infective stages within several weeks. The habitat of adult *Litomosoides carinii* is located in the pleural cavity of cotton rats (*Sigmodon hispidus*). Their sheathed microfilariae are engorged by the mite *Ornithonyssus bacoti.* Owing to their blood-dwelling microfilariae, infections induced by *L. carinii* and by *A. viteae* provide useful models for human lymphatic filariases. The latter is also of interest for the development of vaccines against filarial infections (The Edna McConnel Clark Foundation, 1991). Our third filaria, *Monanema martini,* whose host is the striped mouse *Lemniscomys striatus,* has sheathed skin-dwelling microfilariae. Owing to some pathological features, e. g. the development of skin and eye lesions, this parasite-host system is used as a model for onchocerciasis (Vuong *et al.,* 1991).

The present paper reports on the maintenance of these filarial cycles in the laboratory; it also assesses the efficiency of alternative techniques already available or in preparation, as far as cycle maintenance is concerned.

15.2   Material and Methods

15.2.1   Host animals
The vertebrate hosts *S. hispidus* and *L. striatus* are not commercially available and must therefore be bred in the laboratory. Host animals with uniform biological characteristics are an essential prerequisite for most investigations of the delicate parasite-host interaction; as a result, inbred strains are needed. *M. unguiculatus* was therefore also bred in our laboratory.

15.2.2   Isolation of microfilariae
Skin-dwelling microfilariae of *M. martini* are predominantly located in the ear lobes of striped mice. Small skin biopsies were excised with a corneoscleral punch and incubated in tissue culture medium RPMI 1640 (Bianco *et al.,* 1983). After several hours, most microfilariae had emerged from the biopsies and were transferred to fresh medium. Blood-dwelling microfilariae of *A. viteae* or *L. carinii* were isolated after heparinization of blood taken from the retroorbital vein plexus (Tilgner and Metzke, 1964). Microfilariae of *L. carinii* were purified by density gradient centrifugation over a Percoll gradient (Chandrashekar *et al.,* 1984). The microfilariae of *A. viteae* were separated by agglutination of blood cells with phytohemagglutinin (Wegerhof and Wenk, 1979).

15.2.3   Rearing of the vectors
O. moubata were fed on guinea pigs or rats for about 30 min at monthly or two-monthly intervals. Since the three stages of hard ticks spend several days attached to the host, feeding them under laboratory conditions required special attention. Their final stage were fed on rabbits. The mite *O. bacoti* required regular blood meals at short intervals once or twice a week. Since these tiny arthropods are very agile, blood donors were enclosed in a wire grate for purposes of inactivation. They were then placed directly in the containers harboring the mite colonies, remaining there overnight. Heatable blood chambers originally constructed for artificial

feeding of ceratopogonids, or black flies, were modified to permit feeding at artificial membranes. These chambers were adapted to the feeding habits of mites or ticks, and different blood sources were used (Fahrner and Barthelmess, 1987; Issmer *et al.*, 1994, this volume).

15.2.4   Natural and artificial infestation of the vectors with microfilariae

The different vectors were fed as described above, but this time on infected hosts. To permit a successful infestation, use was made of hosts with a known parasitic load.

The infestation of vectors at membranes was induced by supplementing the blood suspensions in the blood chambers of the feeding apparatus with microfilariae isolated from infected hosts (Issmer *et al.*, 1994, this volume). As with natural infestations, the microfilarial densities of the offered blood meal were decisive in obtaining an adequate yield of infective larvae. Alternatively, the artificial infestation of soft ticks was achieved by inoculating microfilariae into the vector using fine capillary tubes (Weiss *et al.*, 1991).

15.2.5   Isolation of infective larvae and infection of the vertebrate host

Infested vectors were dissected in tissue culture medium RPMI 1640. Infective larvae isolated from mites and hard ticks were taken up directly with a capillary tube. Dissected soft ticks were subsequently transferred to a Bearman funnel in order to separate and purify the infective larvae that emerged from the tissue fragments. Infective larvae were inoculated into the hosts subcutaneously.

15.2.6   Cryopreservation of different stages of the parasite

For the cryopreservation of microfilariae and infective larvae, different types and concentrations of cryoprotectants were tried out. One- or two-step cooling and thawing procedures were applied in order to recover a maximum yield of viable larvae. For the cryopreservation of microfilariae of *L. carinii* we used as standard technique the incubation of microfilariae in RPMI 1640 with 10% dimethylsulfoxide (DMSO) for 5 min, cooling at a rate of 1°/min to $-70\,°C$ and stored in liquid nitrogen. Infective larvae (L3) of *L. carinii* were incubated in RPMI 1640 with 33% polyvinylpyrrolidon (PVP) and 6% DMSO and cooled as described before.

Microfilariae and infective larvae of *A. viteae* were put in RPMI 1640 with 20% fetal calf serum and 9% DMSO on ice, held on ice for a further 10 min and transferred into the vapor phase of liquid nitrogen. They were allowed to stay there for 24 hr and then stored in liquid nitrogen. In a second approach, infective larvae of *A. viteae* were cryopreserved in situ in the vector prior to dissection. Live ticks (*O. moubata*) were cryopreserved in the same way as the microfilariae of *A. viteae*.

15.2.7   In vitro techniques

Microfilariae, infective larvae and adult filariae were cultured using different media and different supplements such as sera, antibiotics or mammalian cells. The physicochemical conditions (e. g. temperature, gas phases, pH and osmolarity) were adapted to the suspected natural conditions (according to Mössinger, 1990).

15.3   Results

15.3.1   Maintenance and infestation of the vector colony

Stable vector populations were obtained when fed on rodents or other small mammals. The number of animals regularly needed for the maintenance of permanent acarine colonies varied considerably depending on the vector and host species. It happened that animals exposed to *O. bacoti* did not survive the procedure of feeding. Death was due to toxicity of saliva or stress, in particular when the number of mites was high. Hosts of *O. moubata* were exposed to the feeding procedure under anesthesia and for short periods only. That might be the main reason why the natural feeding of this tick was accompanied by fewer complications. On the other hand, frequent anesthesia at short intervals could also end fatally for guinea pigs. Rabbits could only be used once or twice as hosts for *H. truncatum* due to immunological reactions to the saliva of the ticks. Low egg deposition and a low rate of larval development were observed when ticks were fed on such immunized rabbits (Fielden *et al.*, 1992).

Alternative feeding techniques using artificial membranes showed differential success depending on the vector species used (Table 15-1). The feeding of *O. moubata* posed no diffi-

Table 15-1. Alternative approaches to replacing the vertebrate hosts of vectors. Grade of feasibility: +++ routine technique, ++ good success, + partial success, – no success, ? not determined.

	Vector		
	O. bacoti	*O. moubata*	*H. truncatum*
Artificial feeding	+++	++	++
Infestation with microfiliariae via membranes	++	++	?
Cryopreservation of			
Eggs	?	?	?
Larvae	?	?	?

culties and likewise mites and hard ticks were successfully fed at membranes. However, it was still not possible to establish stable mite colonies after several bouts of artificial feeding, owing to reduced egg production plus the great agility of these arthropods and the difficulty of handling large numbers of them outside their breeding containers. Although hard ticks need to spend several days attached to their host, the period of attachment of *H. truncatum* on the membranes was long enough for sufficient uptake of blood and subsequent production of eggs (Issmer *et al.*, 1994, this volume).

One to five infective larvae of *L. carinii* per mite were harvested after natural infestation, while up to 20 L3 of *M. martini* per hard tick and up to several hundred L3 of *A. viteae* developed in a single *O. moubata*. All vectors were able to take up microfilariae through the membranes, i.e. the infestation of ticks or mites with microfilariae at artificial membranes proved in principle feasible. Microfilariae of *A. viteae* and, in a few cases, also those of *L. carinii* developed to infective stages.

The intra-abdominal inoculation of microfilariae into the vectors was partially successful as a further alternative approach for obtaining infective larvae. Microfilariae of *A. viteae* injected into the abdomen of *O. moubata* developed to the infective stage. Mites were not subjected to intra-abdominal inoculation of microfilariae due to their small size.

15.3.2   Infection of the hosts

Natural infection achieved very irregular parasitic loads, and complications occurred, as described above for natural feeding. Standardized infections with a well-defined parasitemia could more easily be achieved by quantitative inoculation of infective larvae with a capillary tube than by natural feeding. About 30 to 60 % of *L. carinii* or *A. viteae* and 20 to 50 % of the inoculated larvae of *M. martini* developed to the adult stages. The prepatent phases were completed after eight to ten weeks.

15.3.3   Cryopreservation of parasitic stages

High motility of parasitic stages upon thawing after cryopreservation was a principal criterion for the quality of the cryopreservation. However, not in all cases was a very motile parasite able to undergo further development in the corresponding vector or host. Hence, parasite viability could only be assured when further development could actually be demonstrated. This was observed for isolated cryopreserved infective larvae of *A. viteae*, likewise for *L. carinii* isolated from mites that had been cyropreserved in toto prior to dissection (Table 15-2).

Table 15-2. Availability of alternative methods of maintaining different parasite stages in vitro. Grade of feasibility: +++ routine technique, ++ good success, + partial success, – no success, ? not determined.

	Rodent filaria		
	A. viteae	*L. carinii*	*M. martini*
Microfilariae isolated from the host			
Maintenance in vitro	++	++	++
Development in vitro	–	–	–
Cryopreservation	++	+	++
Infective larvae (vector stages)			
Cryopreservation of			
Isolated L3	++	+	+
L3 in the vector	++	?	++
Infective larvae (vertebrate stages)			
Maintenance in vitro	++	+	+
Development of L4 in vitro	++	–	?
Adult filarial worms			
Maintenance in vitro	++	++	++
Development of intra-uterine stages	+	+	+
Output of microfilaria in vitro	++	+++	+
Cryopreservation	?	?	?

15.3.4   In vitro cultivation of parasitic stages

All stages of the parasite could be maintained in vitro for limited periods (Table 15-2). Microfilariae were able to develop to the late first larva (sausage stage), but not beyond. Infective stages of *L. carinii* and *A. viteae* isolated from the vectors were able to develop to the fourth stage, whereas those of *M. martini* failed to do so. Adult worms survived up to several weeks or months. The intrauterine development of embryonic stages was stunted, thus any release of microfilariae was limited and no reinsemination could be observed.

15.4   Discussion

The establishment and maintenance of filarial cycles in the laboratory is very laborious and their breakdown or loss may be disastrous for research, endangering the work of years. Hence, any alternative techniques for their maintenance need to be not only efficient but also absolutely reliable at the same time. A final logical alternative objective should be the in vitro cultivation of the whole parasitic cycle, completely dispensing with the vertebrate host. However, this is an unrealistic aim going far beyond present feasibilities.

Nevertheless, we were emboldened to develop at least some alternative techniques, substituting short phases of the parasitic cycles only. We had already had good experience with the artificial feeding of ceratopogonids (Fahrner and Barthelmess, 1987), and had found that a permanent colony of *Culicoides nubeculosus* could be maintained without the need for laboratory hosts. Remarkably, membrane feeding of this dipteran ectoparasite turned out to be even more efficient than "natural" feeding on white mice. A rich uptake of blood was not necessarily associated with a subsequent deposition of developing eggs. The reproductivity depended on the source of blood, the quantity of blood engorged, the addition of supplements, possible contamination of the blood meal, etc. We defined a reproductivity index as a reliable indicator of feeding technique efficiency. This factor considered the number of eggs deposited, the rate of hatching of egg larvae, and the development of adults. The envisaged artificial infestation of mites and ticks with microfilariae seems in principle feasible, but it still requires technical improvement and the incorporation of quantitative aspects.

Access to a regular supply of parasitic material (i. e. of viable microfilariae, infective stages or adult worms) is a further prerequisite when conducting many bioassays. This means that a large number of animals have to be infected in order to have sufficient numbers of viable parasites available at any given time. Since the different phases of filarial infection in the vertebrate host operate according to their own dynamics, huge numbers of microfilariae are often available, even when they do not happen to be needed for experimental purposes.

A further decisive step will therefore be the improvement of cryopreservation techniques, so that the presently needed large stocks of infected animals can be reduced or replaced. Viable microfilariae could then be harvested ahead of time and stored till use. Thus, only few infected animals would supply sufficient parasitic material for either assays or cycle maintenance.

A high degree of viability of thawed microfilariae or infective larvae is an essential prerequisite if maintenance of filarial cycles is to be facilitated by "deepfreezing" discrete phases. Since motility alone may give false results, the actual viability of thawed microfilariae and infective stages can be proven in bioassays only, i.e. by challenge of vector and host, respectively. Vectors have to be infested with thawed microfilariae to develop infective stages, while thawed infective stages inoculated into the corresponding vertebrate host must necessarily result in patent infections. Further advanced filarial stages are more difficult to cryopreserve than microfilariae. Since infective stages seem to be rather vulnerable after isolation, it can be speculated that cryopreservation of infective larvae in situ in the living vector, i. e. prior to dissection, would be another very interesting approach. In the vector tissue, parasites are better protected, and there are indications that they might better withstand the taxing procedures of cryopreservation. This possibility is in need of further investigation.

The combination of both techniques, artificial feeding of vectors and the cryopreservation of the parasite, should significantly reduce the number of host animals that are at present still required to maintain the filarial cycle. We estimate that the systematic improvement and consequent application of the alternative techniques presented here will before long permit replacement of more than 50 % of the animals now needed for filarial research, without impairing research quality.

Acknowledgements. We are greatly indebted to Professor Richard Lucius, Hohenheim, who developed the chambers for the feeding of *O. moubata*, and to Mrs. Sofia Theil, Christa Eck and Johanna Backes for excellent technical assistance. Our investigations were supported by the Commission of the European Communities (contract nos. STD2-M-002 and TS 3 CT 91–0037) and the Ministerium für Wissenschaft und Forschung Baden-Württemberg.

References

Bianco A. E., Muller R. and Nelson N. S. (1983) Biology of *Monanema globulosa*, a rodent filaria with skin-dwelling microfilariae. *Journal of Helminthology* **57**, 259–278.

Chandrashekar R., Roa U. R., Rajasekariah G. R. and Subrahmanyam D. (1984) Separation of viable microfilariae free of blood cells on Percoll gradients. *Journal of Helminthology* **58**, 69–70.

The Edna McConnel Clark Foundation (1991) *Strategic plan for onchocerciasis research*. Graphic Center, East Rutherford, N. J. USA

Fahrner J. and Barthelmess C. (1987) Rearing of *Culicoides nubeculosus* (Diptera: Ceratopogonidae) by natural or artificial feeding in the laboratory. *Veterinary Parasitology* **28**, 307–313.

Fahrner J., Vankan D. and Schulz-Key H. (1987) Ingestion of microfilariae from different sources by *Culicoides nubeculosus* (Diptera: Ceratopogonidae) through an artificial membrane. *Veterinary Parasitology* **28**, 315–320.

Fielden L. J., Rechav Y. and Bryson N. R. (1992) Acquired immunity to larvae of *Amblyomma marmoreum* and *A. hebraeum* by tortoises, guinea-pigs and guinea-fowl. *Medical and Veterinary Entomology* **6**, 251–254.

Issmer A. E., Schilling T. H., Vollmer A. and Grunewald, J. (1994) Replacement of laboratory animals in the management of blood-sucking arthropods. In *Alternatives to Animal Testing. New Ways in the Biomedical Sciences, Trends and Progress*. Edited by C. A. Reinhardt. pp. 125–129. VCH Verlagsgesellschaft, Weinheim.

Mössinger J. (1990) Nematoda: Filaroidea. In *In vitro Cultivation of Parasitic Helminths*. Edited by J. D. Smyth. pp. 155–186. CRC Press, Boca Raton.

Tilgner G. and Metzke H. (1964) Die Blutentnahme aus den Venen der Orbita. *Zeitschrift für Versuchstierkunde* **5**, 59–77.

Vuong P. N., Wanji S., Sakka L., Kläger, S. and Bain O. (1991) The murid filaria *Monanema martini*: A model for onchocerciasis. *Annales de Parasitologie Humaine et Comparée* **66**, 109–120.

Wegerhof P. H. and Wenk P. (1979) Studies on acquired resistance of the cotton rat against microfilariae of *Litomosoides carinii*. Effects of single and repeated injections of microfilariae. *Zeitschrift für Parasitenkunde* **60**, 55–64.

Weiss B., Soboslay P. T. and Schulz-Key H. (1991) Entwicklung von infektiösen Larven von Mikrofilarien in *Culicoides nubeculosus*. *Mitteilungen der Österreichischen Gesellschaft für Tropenmedizin und Parasitologie* **13**, 151–158.

World Health Organization (1988) *Report of the Steering Committee of the Scientific Working Group on Filariasis, July 1983 – June 1988.* Unpublished document.

16 Improved Drug Metabolizing Capacity of Hepatocytes Co-Cultured with Epithelial Cells and Maintained in a Perifusion System

Rolf Gebhardt

Summary

The maintenance of co-cultures of hepatocytes with epithelial cell lines in a newly developed perifusion system resulted in prolonged survival of the hepatocytes and enhanced stabilization of the biotransforming capacity. Induction of this capacity by inducers such as phenobarbital and 3-methylcholanthrene was also improved. As demonstrated for lonazolac, this approach rendered it possible to determine the kinetics of drug metabolism under steady-state conditions.

Abbreviations. ECOD = ethoxycoumarin O-deethylase; Lon = lonazolac; MC = 3-methylcholanthrene; PB = phenobarbital.

16.1 Introduction

Rat hepatocytes in primary culture provide a useful in vitro system for studies on the metabolism of xenobiotics, if they are co-cultured with liver epithelial cell lines (Bégué *et al.*, 1984; Guguen-Guillouzo *et al.*, 1983; Wegner *et al.*, 1990). Under these conditions the life span of the cultures is considerably prolonged and normal differentiated functions are well preserved. A few years ago, we described a specialized culture system, named "perifusion," where the culture medium is continuously pumped over the cell monolayer (Gebhardt and Mecke, 1979a). These culture conditions considerably improved the hormonal induction of liver-specific enzymes as well as the metabolic performance of the hepatocytes (Gebhardt, 1991b; Gebhardt and Mecke, 1979a, 1979b).

In the present study, we have combined the advantages of co-cultivation with those of a newly designed perifusion system. A long-term comparison of several enzymatic and metabolic characteristics related to drug metabolism and toxicity was performed in order to show the potential benefit of this approach.

16.2 Materials and methods

16.2.1 Isolation and co-cultivation of hepatocytes

Liver parenchymal cells were isolated from male Sprague-Dawley rats (220 to 280 g) according to Gebhardt *et al.* (1990) and co-cultured with the epithelial cell line RL-ET-14 (passages

Alternatives to Animal Testing. New Ways in the Biomedical Sciences, Trends and Progress.
Reinhardt, C. A. (ed.). 1994. © VCH, Weinheim.

142   R. Gebhardt

25 and 40), as described by Schrode *et al.* (1990) in serum-free Williams medium E. Two hours after the seeding of the hepatocytes (0.625 x 10^6 per ml) on collagen coated glass or plastic supports in the culture chamber of the perifusion system (10 ml, 100 cm²), the epithelioid cells (1.1 x 10^6 per ml) were added and the cultures kept under stationary conditions in the incubator for 24 hr. Then the chamber was connected with the perifusion system described in U. S. A. patent #5,010,014 and European patent #0230223 "module cultivator" (manufactured by IBUK, Königsbronn, FRG) (see Gebhardt and Mecke, 1979a, 1979b). The perifusion received a new batch (100 ml) of serum-free medium (dexamethasone 10^{-7} M) every week. Inductions with phenobarbital (PB, 1 mM) and 3-methylcholanthrene (MC, 0.5 µM) were performed as indicated in the legends to the figures and tables.

16.2.2 Incubation and analytical methods
To probe the capacity of phase-I and phase-II reactions, the model substrate lonazolac (Lon) was infused at a concentration of 10 µM into the culture chamber at a flow rate of 10 ml/hr. Samples of the medium draining from the chamber in the open perifusion mode were taken at different times and analyzed for lonazolac and its metabolites by HPLC as described elsewhere (Gebhardt *et al.*, in press).

Total cellular content of cytochrome P450 and ethoxycoumarin O-deethylase (ECOD) activity were measured as previously described (Gebhardt, 1991b; Gebhardt *et al.*, in press).

16.3   Results

16.3.1   Studies on drug metabolizing enzymes
The content of total cytochrome P450 was compared in stationary and perifusion cultures during a 14-day cultivation period. As shown in Table 16-1, spectrophotometrically detectable P450 was rapidly lost in stationary pure hepatocytes, while perifusion led to a reasonable stabilization. In co-cultures with RL-ET-14 cells, maintenance was considerably improved,

Table 16-1. Comparison of the relative amount of total cytochrome P450 in hepatocytes cultured in different culture systems.

Culture system	Relative amount of total cytochtome P450 (%)[a]				
	Cultivation period (days)				
	1	4	7	10	14
Stationary pure culture	31 ± 6[b]	5 ± 6	4 ± 3	n. d.	n. d.
Perifusion	57 ± 8	45 ± 4	39 ± 6	33 ± 6	24 ± 4
Stationary co-culture	82 ± 7	74 ± 8	65 ± 12	71 ± 9	58 ± 11
Perifused co-culture	81 ± 9	80 ± 10	75 ± 12	79 ± 7	76 ± 8

[a] Total cytochrome P450 content of isolated hepatocytes was set at 100%.
[b] Values represent means ± SD of three assays of cultures.
n. d. = not detectable

but perifusion of these co-cultures resulted in an even better stabilization at about 75 to 80 % of that of freshly isolated hepatocytes over the whole cultivation period.

Comparison of ECOD activities led to similar results (Figure 16-1). In particular, induction of the enzyme activity with a combination of PB and MC during a 48-hr period at different cultivation times showed the same ranking, with perifused co-cultures as the most efficient culture approach.

16.3.2   Studies on drug metabolism

The perifusion system can be used for cultivation in the closed mode (Gebhardt and Mecke, 1979a) or for direct determination of the kinetics of the metabolism of model substrates in the open mode. An example of the latter is shown in Figure 16-2 for Lon, which is hydroxylated to Lon-OH and subsequently converted to Lon-sulfate. As illustrated in Figure 16-2, the concentrations of the mother compound Lon as well as those of its metabolites in the effluent from the culture chamber reached a steady state after about 80 min. After this period, the rate of metabolism could be determined for a defined substrate concentration.

With this experimental design, the capacity of pure and co-cultures maintained under stationary or perifusion conditions could be compared (Table 16-2). As expected, stationary pure hepatocyte cultures lost their metabolic capacity quite rapidly. Hepatocytes maintained in perifusion throughout kept a certain metabolic capacity, but those maintained in co-culture metabolized lonazolac much better at any time during the 14-day period. Again, perifused co-cultures showed the highest metabolic capacity and maintained about 75 % of their initial metabolic rate (Table 16-2). When PB and MC were added to the medium, the same ranking

Table 16-2. Comparison of metabolic rates for lonazolac in pure and co-cultures maintained under stationary or perifusion conditions, with (+) and without (−) PB/MC induction.

Culture system	Induction PB/MC[b]	Production of Lon-OH (pmoles/min)[a]	
		Cultivation period	
		2 days	14 days
Stationary pure culture	—	78 ± 19[c]	n. d.
	+	252 ± 26	n. d.
Perifusion	—	143 ± 21	36 ± 15
	+	318 ± 38	187 ± 22
Stationary co-culture	—	124 ± 24	54 ± 11
	+	337 ± 47	220 ± 28
Perifused co-culture	—	184 ± 34	89 ± 25
	+	392 ± 41	301 ± 57

[a] Hepatocytes were cultured in the respective culture system for the periods indicated, and subsequently, rates of Lon hydroxylation were determined during a 90-min perifusion period in the open mode (as in Figure 16-2) irrespective of the type of cultivation. Rates were calculated per 10^6 cells.
[b] Inducers were present throughout cultivation.
[c] Values represent means ± SD of 3 assays of cultures.
n. d. = not detectable

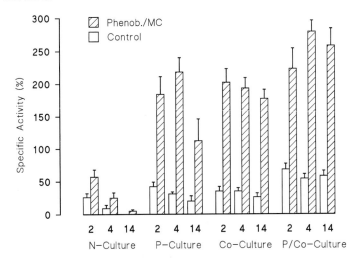

Figure 16-1. Comparison of basal and induced ECOD activities in hepatocytes cultured in different ways. Hepatocytes were maintained in normal (N-Culture), co-culture (Co-Culture), perifusion (P-Culture) or perifused co-culture (P/Co-Culture) for 14 days as in Table 16-1. At the times indicated, samples were taken for measurements of basal and induced ECOD activity. Plates for induction were treated with PB and MC for 48 hr prior to harvesting. ECOD activity in isolated hepatocytes was set at 100%. Values represent means ± SD of three culture assays.

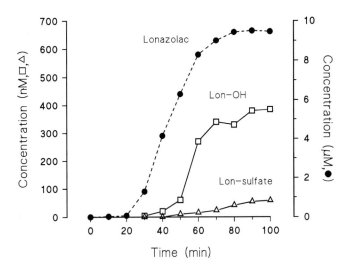

Figure 16-2. Metabolism of lonazolac in perifused co-cultures of hepatocytes determined in the open perifusion system. Hepatocytes in co-culture with RL-ET-14 cells were perifused in the closed mode in the presence of the inducers MC and PB for 48 hr. Then Lon (10 μM) was infused in the open mode for 100 min. Lon and its metabolites were measured in the medium draining from the chamber. Note the establishment of steady-state concentrations in the case of Lon, Lon-OH and Lon-sulfate after 80 min of incubation. Values represent means of duplicate determinations.

order was observed for the induction of lonazolac metabolism (Table 16-2). Under such perifusion conditions, the rates of lonazolac metabolism approached those measured in vivo (Hümpel *et al.*, 1989).

16.4   Discussion

The perifusion of hepatocytes with ordinary serum-free media has a considerable beneficial effect on hepatocyte life span and performance in culture (Gebhardt, 1991a; Gebhardt and Mecke, 1979a, 1979b), although it is somewhat less efficient than co-cultivation with epithelial cell lines. As shown in this paper, the combination of both methods provides even more adequate conditions for the long-term cultivation of metabolically competent hepatocytes, particularly with respect to drug metabolism. This may result from the fact that necessary cell-cell interactions (Mesnil *et al.*, 1987) present in the co-cultures are combined with an optimized supply of nutrients, the stabilization of medium pH, and a better dilution of harmful metabolites, which in stationary cultures may accumulate in the medium (Gebhardt, 1991a, 1991b).

   In addition to an improved performance, there are several other advantages of this culture approach for studies on drug metabolism and cytotoxicity. For instance, hepatocytes in stationary cultures are incubated under non-steady-state conditions, leading to changing concentrations of substrates and products and thus production rates. In contrast, perifusion in the open mode allows the determination of maximal metabolic rates, because steady-state conditions are reached after a certain period of time.

Acknowledgements. This work was supported by the Bundesministerium für Forschung und Technologie and the Landesforschungs-Schwerpunktprogramm Baden-Württemberg.

References

Bégué J. M., Guguen-Guillouzo C., Pasdeloup N. and Guillouzo A. (1984) Prolonged maintenance of active cytochrome P-450 in adult rat hepatocytes co-cultured with another liver cell-type. *Hepatology* **4**, 839–842.

Gebhardt R. (1991a) Histochemical approaches to the screening of carcinogens in vitro. In *Progress in Histo- and Cytochemistry.* Vol. 23. Edited by W. Graumann and J. Drukker. pp. 91–99. Fischer Verlag, Stuttgart, New York.

Gebhardt R. (1991b) Möglichkeiten und Grenzen der Kultivierung von differenzierten Leberparenchymzellen – eine Standortbestimmung. In *Zellkultur in der experimentellen Pathologie.* Edited by E. Schmutzer and G. Neupert. pp. 5–22. Verlagsabteilung der Friedrich-Schiller-Universität, Jena.

Gebhardt R., Alber J., Wegner H. and Mecke D. (in press) Different drug metabolizing capacities in cultured periportal and perivenous hepatocytes. *Biochemical Pharmacology.*

Gebhardt R., Fitzke H., Fausel M., Eisenmann-Tappe I. and D. Mecke (1990) Influence of hormones and drugs on glutathione-S-transferase levels in primary culture of adult rat hepatocytes. *Cell Biology and Toxicology* **6**, 365–378.

Gebhardt R. and Mecke D. (1979a) Perifused monolayer cultures of rat hepatocytes as an improved in vitro system for studies on ureogenesis. *Experimental Cell Research* **124**, 349–359.

Gebhardt R. and Mecke D. (1979b) Permissive effect of dexamethasone on glucagon induction of urea-cycle enzymes in perifused monolayer cultures of rat hepatocytes. *European Journal of Biochemistry* **97**, 29–35.

146   *R. Gebhardt*

Guguen-Guillouzo C., Clement B., Baffet G., Beaumont C., Morel-Chany E., Glaise D. and Guillouzo A. (1983) Maintenance and reversibility of active albumin secretion by adult rat hepatocytes cocultured with another liver epithelial cell type. *Experimental Cell Research* **143**, 47–54.
Hümpel M., Sostarek D., Gieschen H. and Labitzky C. (1989) Studies on the biotransformation of lonazolac, bromerguride, lisuride and terguride in laboratory animals and their hepatocytes. *Xenobiotica* **19**, 361–377.
Mesnil M., Fraslin J. M., Piccoli C., Yamasaki H. and Guguen-Guillouzo C. (1987) Cell contact but not junctional communication (dye coupling) with biliary epithelial cells is required for hepatocytes to maintain differentiated functions. *Experimental Cell Research* **173**, 524–533.
Schrode W., Mecke D. and Gebhardt R. (1990) Induction of glutamine synthetase in periportal hepatocytes by cocultivation with a liver epithelial cell line. *European Journal of Cell Biology* **53**, 35–41.
Wegner H., Mecke D. and Gebhardt R. (1990) The influence of inducing agents and cocultivation on the stability of monooxygenase-activity in rat hepatocyte cultures. *Biological Chemistry Hoppe-Seyler* **371**, 753.

17 Characterization and Use of Long-Term Liver Cultures to Evaluate the Toxicity of Cyclophosphamide or Benzene to Bone Marrow Cultures

Brian A. Naughton, Benson Sibanda, Julia San Román, and Gail K. Naughton

Summary

A method of co-culturing rat hepatic parenchymal cells and liver-derived stromal cells was developed in our laboratory. Hepatocyte co-cultures synthesized albumin, fibrinogen, and other liver-specific proteins and manifested dioxin-inducible cytochrome P450 enzyme activity for ca. 2 months in vitro. The direct effects of alcohols and the chemotherapeutic drugs cytosine arabinoside (Ara-C) and 5-fluorouracil (FU) on viability and ^{3}H-thymidine incorporation into DNA of cultured liver cells were measured. Viability of cultured liver cells, as determined by MTT assay, diminished with increasing doses of methanol, ethanol, or propanol. In addition, Ara-C and FU inhibited DNA synthesis in liver cultures in a dose-related manner. Cyclophosphamide (CP) or benzene was added to flasks containing both dioxin-induced liver cultures and bone marrow (BM) cultures or to BM cultures alone. Hematotoxicity was assessed using flow cytometry, colony forming unit-culture (CFU-C) assay, and neutral red (NR) assay. The presence of metabolically-active hepatocytes exacerbated the toxic effects of CP on BM cultures. Also, at the dose ranges we tested, benzene exerted hematotoxic effects on BM co-cultured with liver but had no discernible effect on BM cultured alone.

Abbreviations. Ara-C = cytosine arabinoside; BM = bone marrow; CFU-C = colony forming unit-culture; CP = cyclophosphamide; EFEE = ethoxyfluorescein ethyl ester; FU = 5-fluorouracil; PC = parenchymal cells.

17.1 Introduction

A variety of chemical agents can induce hematopoietic suppression. This effect is manifested by a defect in the function of a particular blood cell lineage(s), a reduction in the rate of production of certain types of blood cells in bone marrow (BM) or other hematopoietic organs, or both. Assessment of BM toxicity is usually performed in vivo. However, several culture techniques have been used to determine the effects of drugs on hematologic cells. The most common in vitro method measures the effects of drugs on the ability of BM cells to grow into colonies from single cells (called colony forming units, CFU) when plated into defined medium (Beran *et al.*, 1988; Gallichio *et al.*, 1987; Nakarai and Koizumi, 1990). The influence of drugs

Alternatives to Animal Testing. New Ways in the Biomedical Sciences, Trends and Progress.
Reinhardt, C. A. (ed.). 1994. © VCH, Weinheim.

on the response of cultured lymphocytes to phytohemagglutinin (Dornfest *et al.*, 1990) and other mitogens (Chu and Howell, 1981) also has been ascertained. In addition, we (Naughton *et al.*, 1991b, 1992) and others (Williams *et al.*, 1988) have used long-term BM cultures to measure the effects of drugs on hematopoiesis. The putative benefit of long-term BM cultures is that they contain hematopoietic cells as well as BM stromal cells, thereby providing a milieu that resembles the in vivo condition. Stromal cell-associated hematopoiesis was first described by Dexter and co-workers in 1977. Stromal cells secrete hematopoietic growth and regulatory molecules, synthesize specialized matrix for the hematopoietic microenvironment, and have some drug-metabolizing capability (Naughton *et al.*, 1992).

Primary cultures of rat hepatocytes are used routinely to evaluate the influence of potential toxins on enzyme leakage, metabolism, and cellular membrane integrity (Acosta and Mitchell, 1981). In suspension culture, the viability of hepatocytes rapidly declines as does the ability of these cells to manifest inducible cytochrome P450 monooxygenase activity (Sirica and Pitot, 1980), and cell division is limited to the first 24–48 hr of culture (Clayton and Darnell, Jr., 1983). In efforts to enhance the extent and longevity of their metabolic activity in vitro, hepatocytes have been cultured on type I collagen plates and membranes (Michalopoulos and Pitot, 1975), homogenized liver biomatrix (Reid *et al.*, 1980), in collagen type IV or laminin-rich gels (Bissell *et al.*, 1987), sandwiched between two layers of type I collagen (Dunn *et al.*, 1989), on plates coated with fibronectin or other extracellular matrix proteins (Deschenes *et al.*, 1980), and with other cell types (Guguen-Guillouzo *et al.*, 1983; Kuri-Harcuch and Mendoza-Figueroa, 1989; Michalopoulos *et al.*, 1979). The present report describes the long-term expression of cytochrome P450 enzyme activity and albumin production by hepatic parenchymal cells (PC) co-cultured with hepatic stromal cells on nylon screens suspended in liquid medium. The effect of various agents on these liver cell cultures was determined. In addition, BM cultures, either singly or in combination with dioxin-induced liver cultures, were exposed to CP or benzene, and the effects of these agents on hematopoiesis were assessed.

17.2   Materials and Methods

17.2.1   Bone marrow culture

Adult Long-Evans rat BM was used to initiate the cultures (Figure 17-1). The suspended nylon screen BM culture method was described in detail previously (Naughton *et al.*, 1987, 1992; Naughton and Naughton, 1988). Briefly, medullary and endosteal femoral marrow was removed, suspended, and plated in liquid medium. Adherent (stromal) cells were grown for several passes and inoculated onto nylon filtration screens (#3–210/36, Tetko, Inc., NJ). BM hematopoietic cells were inoculated onto the matrix when stromal cell processes spanned most of the mesh openings. Multilineage hematopoiesis develops in a three-dimensional manner within the sieve spaces of this template (Naughton *et al.*, 1987; Naughton and Naughton, 1988).

17.2.2   Liver cultures

Cell isolation

Vascular prograde perfusion of male Long-Evans rat livers was performed in situ as described previously (Naughton *et al.*, 1991a). Liver cell suspensions were passed over a 180-

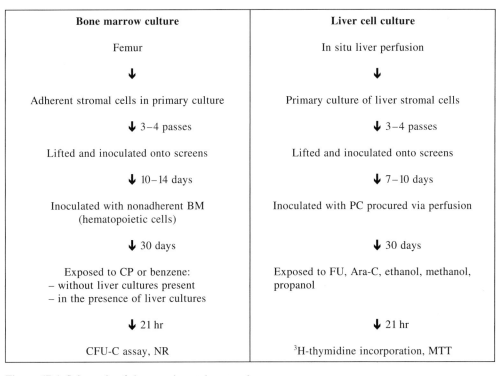

Bone marrow culture	Liver cell culture
Femur	In situ liver perfusion
↓	↓
Adherent stromal cells in primary culture	Primary culture of liver stromal cells
↓ 3–4 passes	↓ 3–4 passes
Lifted and inoculated onto screens	Lifted and inoculated onto screens
↓ 10–14 days	↓ 7–10 days
Inoculated with nonadherent BM (hematopoietic cells)	Inoculated with PC procured via perfusion
↓ 30 days	↓ 30 days
Exposed to CP or benzene: – without liver cultures present – in the presence of liver cultures	Exposed to FU, Ara-C, ethanol, methanol, propanol
↓ 21 hr	↓ 21 hr
CFU-C assay, NR	^{3}H-thymidine incorporation, MTT

Figure 17-1. Schematic of the experimental protocols.

µm filter to remove clumps. Hepatic cells were separated into parenchymal (PC) and stromal (littoral) populations using Percoll gradient centrifugation. To isolate PC, cell suspensions were layered atop a solution of 25% Percoll (Pharmacia Inc., NJ) in 10X Dulbecco's phosphate buffered saline (PBS), centrifuged to remove subcellular debris, washed and resuspended in medium, and centrifuged against a 70% Percoll gradient. The pellet contained a high concentration of PC.

    Hepatic stromal cells consisting of fibroblasts, endothelia, adipocytes, and Kupffer cells were concentrated in the following manner: Freshly isolated cells were centrifuged against a 70% Percoll gradient in 10X PBS (density = 1.09 g/ml) for 10 min forming a pellet and a central zone. Cells from the central zone were washed and centrifuged on a 25%/50% Percoll column. The interface zone (density = 1.03625 g/ml) contained stromal cells, and occasional peripheral blood leukocytes. These cells were plated into liquid culture and their numbers expanded for 3–4 passes.

Culture method
Nylon filtration screens were treated with 1.0 M acetic acid, washed in distilled water, and soaked in fetal bovine serum to enhance cell attachment. These were placed in Tissue Tek slide chambers (Nunc, Inc., IL) and inoculated with 10^7 liver stromal cells which were lifted enzymatically from monolayer culture. Screens were transferred to 25-cm^2 flasks 18–24 hr later. When stromal cells extended processes across most of the mesh openings the templates

were inoculated with 2–5 x 10^6 hepatic PC and transferred to 25-cm^2 flasks after 18–24 hr. Cells were cultured (5 % CO_2, 35–37 °C, >90 % humidity) in DMEM conditioned with 6 % fetal bovine serum and 10 % equine serum and supplemented with 70 μg glucagon (Sigma #G9261), 5 mg insulin (Sigma #I4011), 0.25 mg glucose, and 231 μg hydrocortisone hemi-succinate per 500 ml of medium. Complete medium replacement was performed 5 times per week.

17.2.3   Methods of evaluation

Albumin assay

Medium was collected during each feeding and tested for the presence of rat albumin using the enzyme-linked immunosorbent assay (ELISA) (Dunn *et al.*, 1989). Chromatographically pure rat albumin and peroxidase-conjugated anti-rat albumin were purchased from Cappel Inc. (PA) and absorbance at 490 nm was determined using a kinetic microplate reader (Molecular Devices Inc., CA). 100 μl of spent medium was added to 96-well plates and stored at 0 °C for 12–14 hr. The wells were washed with 0.5 % Tween-20 in PBS and non-specific binding sites were blocked with 5.0 % BSA in PBS. After washing with 0.5 % Tween-20, 100 μl of sheep anti-rat albumin-peroxidase conjugate was added to each well and incubated (1 hr, 22 °C). The wells were washed with 0.5 % Tween-20 and incubated for 15 min with *o*-phenylenediamine substrate (Cappel Inc., PA). The reaction was stopped and absorbance was measured on an EIA reader.

Cytochrome P450 assay

Freshly isolated hepatocytes, hepatocytes 24 hr after isolation, and hepatocytes derived from suspended nylon screen cultures of various durations were assayed for cytochrome P450 monooxygenase activity by flow cytometry. One nM of a 1-μM stock solution of 2,3,7,8-tetrachlorodibenzo-*p*-dioxin (TCDD) (Chemical Carcinogen Repository, National Cancer Institute, MO) in dimethylsulfoxide (DMSO) (Sigma Chem. Co.) was added to cell cultures for 18 hr to induce enzyme activity (Miller, 1983). This non-fluorescent compound was found to be an ideal inducer for this assay. Cells in suspended nylon screen cultures were lifted using dispase-collagenase, pelleted and resuspended in PBS at a density of ca. 5 x 10^5 cells/ml, stored on ice for 1 hr, and gradually warmed to 37 °C. Cells were analyzed for evidence of cytochrome P450 enzyme activity by quantifying incremental fluorescein fluorescence in cells accumulating ethoxyfluorescein ethyl ester (EFEE) (Miller, 1983; White *et al.*, 1987). Cells were incubated with 50 nM EFEE (Molecular Probes, Eugene, OR) in PBS for 5 min at 37 °C and examined for green fluorescence on a flow cytometer with a 515-nm long-pass filter and tuned to the 488 nm band. Fluorescence was gated on various populations of cells based on differences in forward light scatter versus side scatter characteristics and was measured once per minute for up to 15 min in samples maintained at 37 °C. Fluorescein accumulation in cells over time was indicative of cytochrome P450 activity.

Viability assays

Intact BM or liver cultures were cut into 8 mm x 10 mm pieces and placed in 24-well plates. After drug treatment, the cultures were washed in complete medium and re-incubated for 24 hr (35 °C, 5 % CO_2). Cultures were incubated for 12 hr in DMEM with 2 % FBS and either 50 μg/ml neutral red (Borenfreund and Peurner, 1984) or 0.5 mg/ml MTT (Carmichael *et al.*, 1987) (Sigma Chemical Co., MO). The dye incorporated by viable cells was extracted with solvent and the optical density of the medium at 540 nm was measured with a kinetic micro-plate reader (Molecular Devices Corp., CA). Results were plotted as percentage of untreated controls (ratio of OD_{540} test to OD_{540} control x 100).

CFU-C assay
Our procedure was a modification of the method of Bradley and Metcalf (1966) for culturing colonies containing myeloid and monocytic cells in agar with defined medium. It has been described in detail previously (Naughton *et al.*, 1991b, 1992). CFU-culture (C) is a parameter that measures the proliferative capacity of BM cells.

Radiothymidine incorporation
^{3}H-thymidine was added to 10 mm x 10 mm pieces of liver cultures in 24-well plates at a con-centration of 1 µCi/well, and the cultures were incubated at 5 % CO_2. After 24 hr, the medium was removed and cells were dissociated from the screens with collagenase/dispase, pelleted at 200 g, washed, and lysed for protein precipitation with trichloroacetic acid (30-min treat-ment, 4 °C). Precipitate was harvested onto a glass fiber filter and ^{3}H-thymidine incorporation was read with a Betaplate scintillation counter (Pharmacia, Finland).

Drug treatment
Liver cultures were induced with dioxin, cut into 8 mm x 10 mm pieces and placed into 24-well plates with BM cultures of equal dimensions. The two cultures were separated by a blank nylon screen with 180-µm sieve openings and CP (0–0.1%) or benzene (0–10^4 ppm) were introduced into the system. After 21 hr, the BM cultures were removed and either assayed for viability using the MTT method or treated with enzyme and assayed for CFU-C content.

The effect of various levels of ethanol, propanol, or methanol on the viability of 45-day-old liver cultures was determined using the neutral red viability assay.

17.3   Results

Parenchymal cells that were cultured on suspended nylon screen/liver stroma templates remained viable and synthesized albumin at levels equal to or greater than that of input cells for 48 days in culture (Figure 17-2). Cells in these co-cultures also exhibited inducible cyto-chrome P450 enzyme activity for up to 58 days as indicated by their ability to transform EFEE to fluorescein (Figure 17-3). This conversion was intracellular since the fluorescence mea-surements were gated on discrete populations of cells identified by their forward light scatter and 90° light scatter characteristics. Highest fluorescence was observed in the larger PC. Arbitrary conversion units were calculated as the product of the percent positive fluorescence and peak channel number as described by Miller (1983). Peak EFEE to fluorescein conversion was higher in the various co-cultures than in either freshly isolated liver cells or 1-day-old suspension cultures of isolated hepatocytes (Figure 17-3). Treatment of liver cultures with alcohols resulted in a dose-related decrease in viability (Figure 17-4), and ^{3}H-thymidine incorporation into DNA of these cultured cells decreased in response to increasing doses of Ara-C and FU (Table 17-1).

Benzene, at exposure levels of 0 to 10^4 ppm, did not exert significant toxicity to BM cul-tures. However, when BM cultures were co-incubated with liver cultures at the time of exposure, a substantial diminution in MTT-assayed viability was observed with benzene levels exceeding 400 ppm (Figure 17-5). The effect of CP exposure to BM in combined BM/liver cultures was more difficult to assess, since some elements of the BM stromal cell population have the ability to convert EFEE to fluorescein (Naughton *et al.*, 1992). Direct treatment of BM cultures with CP resulted in dose related decreases in CFU-C progenitor proliferation and the absolute numbers of hematologic cells in the adherent zones of the suspended nylon screen cultures (Table 17-2). This effect, however, was exacerbated in BM cultures that were exposed to CP when liver cultures were present.

Table 17-1. Mean ^{3}H-thymidine incorporation into DNA (expressed as counts per minute, cpm) of cultured liver cells ($\pm$ SEM) after exposure to various doses of 5 fluorouracil (FU) or cytosine arabinoside (Ara-C).

Dose of FU (mg/ml)	Mean cpm $\pm$ SEM	Dose of Ara-C (mg/ml)	Mean cpm $\pm$ SEM
0	2412 $\pm$ 500	0	8009 $\pm$ 420
0.1	3224 $\pm$ 352	0.5	2200 $\pm$ 376
0.5	2620 $\pm$ 270	1.0	2433 $\pm$ 294
1.0	1816 $\pm$ 212	2.0	900 $\pm$ 130
1.5	1408 $\pm$ 176	3.0	930 $\pm$ 202
2.0	880 $\pm$ 121		

Table 17-2. Effect of cyclophosphamide or benzene on mean numbers of CFU-C per 10^5 cells ($\pm$ 1 SEM) in freshly isolated BM nonadherent cells (without stroma), 30-day-old nylon screen BM cultures, and 30-day nylon screen BM cultures with liver cultures present during drug exposure.

Drug-dose	CFU-C		
	BM nonadherent cells	30-day BM culture	30-day BM culture with liver culture
Cyclophosphamide			
0%	640 $\pm$ 78	576 $\pm$ 55	612 $\pm$ 67
0.025%	589 $\pm$ 70	534 $\pm$ 21	511 $\pm$ 34
0.05%	616 $\pm$ 45	481 $\pm$ 43	408 $\pm$ 53
0.50%	632 $\pm$ 36	297 $\pm$ 60	103 $\pm$ 13
1.00%	618 $\pm$ 26	254 $\pm$ 40	52 $\pm$ 9
Benzene			
0 ppm	–	609 $\pm$ 41	652 $\pm$ 46
1000 ppm	–	617 $\pm$ 61	601 $\pm$ 29
2000 ppm	–	578 $\pm$ 37	540 $\pm$ 41
4500 ppm	–	599 $\pm$ 33	482 $\pm$ 25
10000 ppm	–	569 $\pm$ 28	294 $\pm$ 18

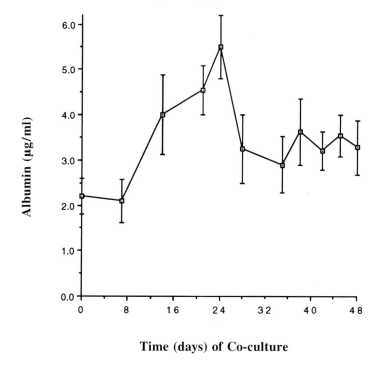

Time (days) of Co-culture

Figure 17-2. Mean albumin levels ($\pm$ SEM) in the spent medium of suspended nylon screen liver cultures as determined by ELISA.

17.4   Discussion

The viability and enzymatic activity of cultured hepatic parenchyma can be prolonged in vitro if the cells are co-cultured with non-parenchymal liver cells, support cells from other tissues, or their products. PC proliferation, however, is limited or absent in these systems. Cytokines originating from these support cells and/or their matrix are necessary for the maintenance of PC cytochrome P450 enzyme activity. In addition, the ability to maintain hepatic PC in culture, even in a mitotically quiescent state, is important to assess the long-term effects of various agents on these cells (Bissell *et al.*, 1987; Guguen-Guillouzo *et al.*, 1983; Michalopoulos and Pitot, 1975). The presence of endothelial cells enhances the ability of human (Begue *et al.*, 1983) or rat (Ratanasavanh *et al.*, 1988) PC to metabolize xenobiotics. In addition, non-hepatic fibroblasts, or extracellular matrix proteins also could extend liver-specific enzyme functions in vitro. In the present study, liver stroma consisting of Kupffer cells (verified by their ability to phagocytose colloidal carbon), vascular endothelial cells (based on recognition by anti-vW f VIII antibody), and biliary endothelia, fibroblasts, and fat cells (identified morphologically) exhibited the ability to support PC function. It may be important when developing culture substrates for toxicity assessments to include all of the relevant cell types found in the system(s) to be studied.

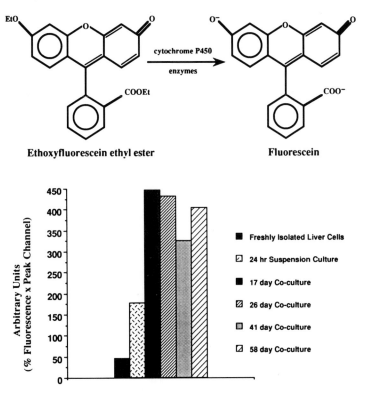

Figure 17-3. Graph depicting mean cytochrome P450 activity in fresh liver cell isolates, a 24-hr-old suspension culture, and suspended nylon screen cultures of various ages. The molecular structures of ethoxyfluorescein ethyl ester and fluorescein are depicted as well.

Co-cultures of liver PC and hepatic stroma on nylon screens exhibit a broad range of liver-specific function including dioxin-inducible cytochrome P450 enzyme activity (Figure 17-3), albumin synthesis (Figure 17-2), and the production of transferrin, fibrinogen, fibronectin, transforming growth factor β, and laminin (data not shown). Although the influence of toxicants on the synthesis of these proteins has not yet been evaluated, suspended nylon screen liver cultures respond in a dose-related fashion to increasing concentrations of alcohols (viability; Figure 17-4) and two chemotherapeutic drugs (DNA synthesis; Table 17-1). The results obtained when liver and BM were co-cultured at the time of exposure to CP or benzene indicated that the liver cultures bioactivated these compounds resulting in a decrease in viability and hematopoietic progenitor activity in the BM cultures.

Conceivably, cultures of other tissues could be substituted for BM in this model system. Although macrophages have been reported to possess cytochrome P450 enzyme activity (Naughton *et al.*, 1992; Santos *et al.*, 1985; Thomas *et al.*, 1990), the EFEE to fluorescein conversion described herein was identified in the largest cells found in the liver cultures. Since PC are ca. twice the size of Kupffer cells, these cells are almost certainly parenchymal in nature.

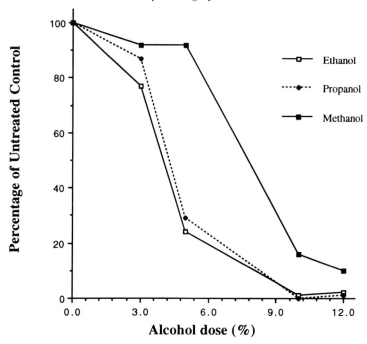

Figure 17-4. Mean percent viability of liver cultures exposed to various concentrations of alcohols as determined by the MTT assay.

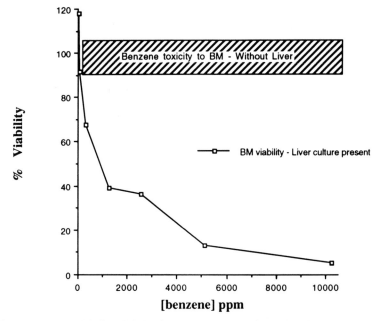

Figure 17-5. Mean percent viability of BM cultures exposed to different levels of benzene with (line) and without (horizontal bar = mean ± SEM) the presence of liver cultures. NR assay.

At the 1990 INVITOX meeting, we reported that CP, which requires activation to its toxic metabolites by enzymes of the cytochrome P450 system (Santos *et al.*, 1985), inhibited hematopoiesis in suspended nylon screen BM cultures (Naughton *et al.*, 1991b). In a recent study, we found that the macrophage subpopulation of BM stroma displayed cytochrome P450 enzyme activity (Naughton *et al.*, 1992), which evidently was responsible for this phenomenon. Two characteristics of long-term BM cultures may act in concert to produce this effect: a) The BM stroma in these cultures is macrophage-rich, and b) developing hematopoietic cells are nourished by macrophages and are found in close apposition to these cells. The generation of even small amounts of radicals by macrophages should induce toxicity in the satellite hematopoietic cells. BM stromal cells also have been reported to metabolize benzene derivatives (Thomas *et al.*, 1990), although we were not able to demonstrate cytotoxicity to our BM cultures using this compound, at least at doses up to 10^4 ppm.

In conclusion, suspended nylon screen cultures exhibit a number of liver-specific functions including long-term expression of inducible cytochrome P450 enzyme activity. These liver cultures can be used for hepatotoxicity measurements and also to bioactivate xenobiotics in co-culture conditions, to assess drug effects on BM and potentially, other target cultures.

References

Acosta D. and Mitchell D. B. (1981) Metabolic activation and cytotoxicity of cyclophosphamide in primary cultures of postnatal rat hepatocytes. *Biochemical Pharmacology* 30, 3225–3231.

Begue J. M., LeBigot J. F., Guguen-Guillouzo C., Kiechel J. R. and Guillouzo A. (1983) Cultured human hepatocytes: a new model for drug metabolism studies. *Biochemical Pharmacology* 32, 1643–1651.

Beran M., Andersson B. S., Wang Y., McCredie K. B. and Farquhar D. (1988) The effects of acetaldophosphamide, a novel stable aldophosphamide analog, on normal human and leukemic progenitor cells *in vitro. Cancer Research* 48, 339–345

Bissell D. M., Arenson D. M., Maher J. J. and Roll J. (1987) Support of cultured hepatocytes by a laminin-rich gel: Evidence for a functionally significant subendothelial matrix in normal rat liver. *Journal of Clinical Investigation* 79, 801–814.

Borenfreund E. and Puerner J. A. (1984) A simple quantitative method using monolayer cultures for cytotoxicity assays. *Journal of Tissue Culturing Methods* 9, 7–9.

Bradley T. R. and Metcalf D. (1966) The growth of mouse bone marrow cells *in vitro. Australian Journal of Experimental Biology and Medical Science* 44, 287–300.

Carmichael J., DeGraff W. G., Gazdar A. F., Minna J. D. and Mitchell J. B. (1987) Evaluation of a tetrazolium-based semiautomated colorimetric assay: assessment of chemosensitivity testing. *Cancer Research* 47, 936–943.

Chu B. C. F. and Howell S. B. (1981) Differential toxicity of carrier-bound methotrexate toward human lymphocytes, marrow, and tumor cells. *Biochemical Pharmacology* (Oxford) 30, 2545–2552.

Clayton R. and Darnell J. E., Jr. (1983) Changes in liver-specific compared to common gene transcription during primary culture of mouse hepatocytes. *Molecular and Cellular Biology* 3, 1552–1561.

Deschenes J., Vale J. P and Marceau, N. (1980) Hepatocytes from newborn and weanling rats in monolayer culture: Isolation by perfusion, fibronectin-mediated adhesion, spreading, and functional activities. *In Vitro* 16, 722–735.

Dexter T. M., Allen T. D. and Lajtha L. G. (1977) Conditions controlling the proliferation of haematopoietic stem cells *in vitro. Journal of Cellular Physiology* 91, 335–344.

Dornfest B. S., Bush M. E., Lapin D. M., Adu S., Fulop A. and Naughton B. A. (1990) Phenylhydrazine is a mitogen and activator of lymphoid cells. *Annals of Clinical and Laboratory Science* 20, 353–361.

Dunn J. C. Y., Yarmush M. L., Koebe H. G. and Tompkins R. G. (1989) Hepatocyte function and extracellular matrix geometry: long-term culture in a sandwich configuration. *The FASEB Journal* **3**, 174–178.

Gallichio V., Casale G. P. and Watts T. (1987) Inhibition of human bone marrow derived stem cell colony formation (CFU-E, BFU-E, and CFU-GM) following *in vitro* exposure to organophosphates. *Experimental Hematolology* **15**, 1099–1103.

Guguen-Guillouzo C., Clement B., Baffet G., Beaumont C., Morel-Chany E., Glaise D. and Guillouzo A. (1983) Maintenance and reversibility of active albumin secretion by adult rat hepatocytes co-cultured with another cell type. *Experimental Cell Research* **143**, 47–54.

Kuri-Harcuch W. and Mendoza-Figueroa T. (1989) Cultivation of adult rat hepatocytes on 3T3 cells: expression of various liver differentiated functions. *Differentiation* **41**, 148–156.

Michalopoulos G. and Pitot H. C. (1975) Primary culture of parenchymal liver cells on collagen membranes. *Experimental Cell Research* **94**, 70–78.

Michalopoulos G., Russel F. and Biles C. (1979) Primary cultures of hepatocytes on human fibroblasts. *In Vitro* **15**, 796–801.

Miller A. G. (1983) Ethylated fluoresceins: Assay of cytochrome P450 activity and application to measurements in single cells by flow cytometry. *Analytical Chemistry* **133**, 46–57.

Nakarai T. and Koizumi S. (1990) Effects of calcium antagonists on anti-cancer drug toxicity to haematopoietic progenitor cells in normal human bone marrow. *Leukemia Research* **14**, 401–405.

Naughton B. A. and Naughton G. K. (1988) Hematopoiesis on nylon screen templates: Modulation of long-term bone marrow culture by stromal support cells. *Annals of the New York Academy of Sciences* **554**, 125–140.

Naughton B. A., Preti R. A. and Naughton G. K. (1987) Hematopoiesis on nylon mesh templates. I. Long-term culture of rat bone marrow cells. *Journal of Medicine: Clinical, Experimental and Theoretical* **18**, 219–250.

Naughton B. A., Sibanda B., Azar L. and San Roman J. (1992) Differential effects of drugs upon hematopoiesis can be assessed in long-term bone marrow cultures established on nylon screens. *Proceedings of the Society for Experimental Biology and Medicine* **199**, 481–490.

Naughton B. A., Sibanda B. and Naughton G. K. (1991a) Long-term liver cell cultures as potential substrates for toxicity assessment, In *Alternative Methods in Toxicology, Vol. 8. In Vitro Toxicology: Mechanisms and New Technology*. Edited by A. M. Goldberg. pp. 193–202. Mary Ann Liebert Publishers, New York.

Naughton B. A., Sibanda B., Triglia D. and Naughton G. K. (1991b) Rat bone marrow cell proliferation as an index of the effects of xenobiotics in vitro. *Toxicology In Vitro* **5**, 389–394.

Ratanasavahn D., Baffet G., Latinier M. F., Rissel, M. and Guillouzo, A. (1988) Use of hepatocyte co-cultures in the assessment of drug toxicity from chronic exposure. *Xenobiotica* **18**, 765–774.

Reid L. M., Gaitmaitan Z., Arias I., Ponce P. and Rojkind M. (1980) Long-term cultures of normal rat hepatocytes on liver biomatrix. *Annals of the New York Academy of Sciences* **349**, 70–81.

Santos M. J., Ojeda J. M., Garrido J. and Leighton F. (1985) Peroxisomal organization in normal and cerebrohepatorenal (Zellweger) syndrome fibroblasts. *Proceedings of the National Academy of Sciences of the United States of America* **82**, 6556–6560.

Sirica A. E. and Pitot H. C. (1980) Drug metabolism and effects of carcinogens in cultured hepatic cells. *Pharmacological Reviews* **31**, 205–223.

Thomas D. J., Sadler A., Subrahmanyam V. V., Siegel D., Reasor M. J., Wierda D. and Ross, D. (1990) Bone marrow stromal cell bioactivation and detoxification of the benzene metabolite hydroquinone: comparison of macrophages and fibroblastic cells. *Molecular Pharmacology* **37**, 255–262.

White I. N. H., Green M. L. and Legg R. F. (1987) Fluorescence-activated sorting of rat hepatocytes based on their mixed function oxidase activities towards diethoxyfluorescein. *Biochemical Journal* **247**, 23–28.

Williams L. H., Udupa K. B. and Lipschitz D. A. (1988) Long-term bone marrow culture as a model for host toxicity: The effect of methotrexate on hematopoiesis and adherent layer function. *Experimental Hematology* **16**, 80–87.

18 European Interlaboratory Evaluation of an in Vitro Ocular Irritation Model (Skin²™ Model ZK1100) Using 18 Chemicals and Formulated Products

Peter W. Joller, Alain Coquette, Jos Noben, Raffaella Pirovano, Jacqueline A. Southee, and Pamela K. Logemann

Summary

To evaluate potential irritancy, four European toxicology laboratories analyzed 18 standardized test substances utilizing three different quantifiable endpoints to Skin²™ cells and tissue supernatants: a) reduction in the total number of viable cells using an MTT assay, b) induction of an inflammatory mediator using PGE_2 measurements, and c) cell membrane damage using LDH release. Three test materials were chosen from each of the following categories: shampoos, alcohols, raw surfactants, metal chlorides, preservatives, and solvents. Qualitative ocular irritation scores (in vivo) were obtained for each of the materials and compared with the quantitative in vitro scores, PGE_2 release, and LDH release. Within each chemical group, the MTT_{50} scores ranked the test materials the same as the ocular irritation scores. For example, the irritation order of baby shampoo < soft shampoo < dandruff shampoo was found both in vivo and in vitro. Similarly, both tests ranked the alcohols in the order, methanol < isopropanol < 1-pentanol; the surfactants in the order Tween 20 < Triton X-100 < benzalkonium chloride; the metal chlorides in the order magnesium chloride < nickel chloride < cadmium chloride; and the preservatives in the order; benzoic acid < imidazolidinyl urea < propylene glycol. The corresponding levels of PGE_2 and LDH release will also be presented.

Abbreviations. DMSO = dimethyl sulfoxide; LDH = lactate dehydrogenase; MTT = dimethylthiazolyl-diphenyltetrazolium bromide; PGE_2 = prostaglandin E_2.

18.1 Introduction

The necessity of in vitro alternatives for irritation studies is obvious and clear. Less clear is the possible way of setting up a reliable and reproducible model to substitute for in vivo animal experiments. The alternative in vitro system should be at least as dependable as the Draize eye irritation test. But going beyond the basic idea requires not only development and validation, but also the creation of acceptability.

To study these questions, Advanced Tissue Sciences together with Janssen Biotech set up a European interlaboratory evaluation study with four contract laboratories: ANAWA, Wangen, Switzerland; RBM, Ivrea, Italy; Microbiological Associates, Inc., Sterling, Scotland (MA); and Laboratoires J. Simon, Wavre, Belgium (SIMON).

Alternatives to Animal Testing. New Ways in the Biomedical Sciences, Trends and Progress.
Reinhardt, C. A. (ed.). 1994. © VCH, Weinheim.

The goal of this study was to test the Skin[2TM] Model ZK 1100 (Braa *et al.*, 1991), which has the following advantages:

– human origin
– three-dimensional, multilayered tissue
– active metabolism
– short-term test (24 hr)
– safe
– quantitative, not only qualitative results
– multiple simultaneous endpoints
– highly standardized manufacturing
– extensively tested in the U.S.A.
– adapted for pharmaceutics, cosmetics, household products
– adapted for chemical compounds, raw materials, and formulated products

The study was set up to evaluate inter- and intralaboratory variations. On two occasions 18 standardized test materials were analyzed by all four laboratories, and for each substance three endpoints were quantitatively determined. In the two independent experiments, two different lots of Skin[2TM] substrate were used.

The in vitro results were compared with the in vivo results using the Draize primary eye irritation test results (OECD guideline No. 405), generated in one of the contract laboratories (SIMON).

18.2   Materials and Methods

Skin[2TM] Model ZK 1100 (Advanced Tissue Sciences Inc., La Jolla, CA) was shipped to Europe by Federal Express to the different laboratory sites and immediately processed. The kit supplies the tissue substrates immersed in an agarose-medium in a 24-well foil-sealed tray. Validated procedure leaflets, culture medium, assay medium, and all disposable, sterile labware is also contained in the kit.

Three endpoints had to be quantified during this study. Dimethylthiazolyl-diphenyl-tetrazolium bromide (MTT) measures the reduction of a tetrazolium salt to insoluble blue formazan by mitochondrial succinic dehydrogenase and serves as an indicator of cell-relevant function damage and cell viability. Lactate dehydrogenase (LDH) released into the culture medium is a measure of membrane damage. Prostaglandin E_2 (PGE_2) is an indicator of irritative effects. MTT, LDH and PGE_2 test kits were also supplied by Advanced Tissue Sciences.

The chemicals and formulated products to be analyzed were selected and distributed by Janssen Biotech. The reference substances were chosen as representatives of six classes of chemicals and formulated products:

Shampoo (100, 300, 700, 1000, 3000 µg/ml)
– Baby shampoo
– Soft shampoo
– Medicated shampoo

Alcohol (0.1, 0.3, 1.0, 3.0, 10.0% v/v)
- Methanol
- Isopropanol
- 1-Pentanol

Raw Surfactants (1, 10, 100, 1000, 10 000 µg/ml)
- Tween 20
- Triton X-100
- Benzalkonium chloride

Metal Chlorides (30, 100, 300, 1000, 3000 µg/ml)
- Magnesium chloride
- Nickel chloride
- Cadmium chloride

Preservatives (1, 10, 100, 1000, 10 000 µg/ml)
- Benzoic acid
- Imidazolidinyl urea
- Propylene glycol

Solvents (0.1, 0.3, 1.0, 3.0, 10.0% v/v)
- Dimethyl sulfoxide (DMSO)
- Acetone
- Xylene

Each compound was dissolved and/or diluted in assay medium according to the above indicated dose range.

According to the test protocol, the 24-well plates received 2 ml of assay medium (negative control) or of each test agent concentration. The substrate Skin²™ tissues were transferred from the shipping tray to each well. Each point was determined in duplicate. Six additional wells were filled with assay medium and blank nylon supports (no cells) to verify any unspecific binding.

The exposure period of the cells was 16 hr in a humidified CO_2 incubator at 37°C. At the end of the culture, the medium was collected from each well and stored at -70°C until performing the LDH assay (Kit LK-100, Protein International) or the assay for PGE_2 (EIA Kit 6801, Advanced Magnetics, Cambridge, U. S. A.). The MTT assay was carried out with the MTT ZA0014 kit (Advanced Tissue Sciences). One ml of MTT solution at 0.5 mg/ml was put into each well, and the plates were incubated for 2 hr at 37°C under continuous shaking. The solution was discarded, the tissue washed twice with saline, and finally the blue formazan extracted with isopropanol (1 ml per well). Reading was done at 540 nm. MTT reduction percentage was calculated in comparison with the untreated controls. For result comparison the OD_{50} values were determined. The entire assay can be finished within 24 hr.

The Draize eye irritation test was performed according to the OECD guideline No. 405. Briefly, rabbits without existing eye defects were used. 100 µl of the test substance in one safe concentration was administered to the conjunctiva of one eye. The upper and the lower eyelid were then carefully closed and held together for 1 s to prevent loss of material. The other eye,

Table 18-1. MTT$_{50}$ values of 18 substances obtained in two separate runs of the Skin^{2TM} (Model ZK1100) assay in four different laboratories.

Test substances	MA		SIMON		RBM		ANAWA	
	1st	2nd	1st	2nd	1st	2nd	1st	2nd
Baby shampoos (µg/ml)								
Baby shampoo	1740	914	1643	911	1630	1830	1701	1507
Soft shampoo	242	202	419	287	410	445	452	377
Med. shampoo	314	366	393	394	420	440	355	315
Alcohols (% v/v)								
Methanol	>10	>10	>10	>10	>10	>10	>10	>10
Isopropanol	5.4	5.3	2.3	2.1	2.6	3.1	4.2	1.9
1-Pentanol	0.57	0.49	0.29	0.24	0.51	0.50	0.41	0.54
Raw surfactants (µg/ml)								
Tween 20	301	283	318	380	320	900	376	375
Triton X-100	25.9	30.5	33.0	33.0	25.5	27.5	28.0	26.8
Benzalk. chl.	1.5	2.6	4.1	3.4	2.7	2.7	2.8	3.5
Metal chlorides (µg/ml)								
Magnesium	>3000	>3000	>3000	>3000	>3000	>3000	>3000	>3000
Nickel	1390	1140	987	1086	1250	720	1050	1240
Cadmium	44	114	44	44	43	44	102	45
Preservatives (µg/ml)								
Benzoic acid	>10000	2950	2600	3176	3250	3100	>10000	2704
Imidaz. urea	25.8	177	285	223	255	230	250	231
Propylene glyc.	—	>10000	>10000	>10000	>10000	>10000	>10000	>10000
Solvents (% v/v)								
DMSO	>10	5.49	>10	>10	>10	>10	>10	>10
Acetone	4.3	5.0	8.4	9.3	>10	>10	4.9	5.3
Xylene	0.14	0.26	6.9	1.8	1.8	5.2	0.52	1.7

remaining untreated, served as control. The test eye was not rinsed out following the adminis-tration of the substance. The eyes were examined at 1, 24, 48, 72, and 96 hr. Ocular reactions were judged as described in the *Journal officièl de la République Française* (24.10.84). Residual eye effects were recorded at weekly intervals in order to allow a proper evaluation of the reversibility of the effects observed.

18.3   Results and Discussion

Table 18-1 shows the MTT_{50} results for each of the two experimental runs in each lab. The values were very similar both intra- and interlaboratory. The only discrepancies occurred with cadmium chloride, xylene, and benzoic acid. Explanations for these divergences were interference of the two former substances with the plastic of the culture vessels and the in-solubility of the latter at the highest concentration resulting in inhomogenous suspensions.

The comparison of the MTT_{50} values, determined in vitro, with the in vivo score of irri-tancy is given in Table 18-2.

Table 18-2. Comparison of in vivo eye irritance (Draize test) with in vitro Skin²ᵀᴹ Model ZK1100.

Test substances	In vivo score[a]	Reversibility after 14 days	In vitro $MTT_{50} \pm SD$
Shampoos			
Baby shampoo	2	–	1484.50 ± 365.02
Soft shampoo	6	yes	354.25 ± 97.04
Medicated shampoo	6	yes	374.63 ± 45.88
Alcohols			
Methanol	8	yes	>10
Isopropanol	26	yes	3.36 ± 1.42
1-Pentanol	28	no	0.44 ± 0.12
Raw surfactants			
Tween 20	0	–	406.63 ± 202.79
Triton X-100	25	no	28.78 ± 3.02
Benzalkonium chloride	87	no	2.91 ± 0.77
Metal chlorides			
Magnesium	0	yes	>3000
Nickel	0	yes	1107.88 ± 202.54
Cadmium	0	yes	60.00 ± 29.80
Preservatives			
Benzoic acid	8	yes	2963.33 ± 262.88
Imidazolidinyl urea	8	yes	209.60 ± 80.43
Propylene glycol	8	yes	>10000
Solvents			
DMSO	8	yes	9.44 ± 1.59
Acetone	12	yes	7.15 ± 2.50
Xylene	16	yes	2.29 ± 2.46

[a] Scored according to OECD guideline 405 from 0 to 100.

Comparison of the in vivo with the in vitro findings shows only differences which are attributable to a too low concentration of the metal chlorides in the Draize test. All other test material is ranked the same way in vivo as in vitro by the MTT test. Not only was there an excellent correlation between the Draize and MTT tests, but also intralaboratory analysis revealed only 3 discrepancies, while minor interlaboratory differences were found in only 4 out of 18 data sets due to close MTT_{50} values and due to the problems with solubility and interference with the labware as stated above. The only unexplained difference between in vivo and in vitro tests was with propylene glycol showing no toxic or irritating properties in the in vitro assay, while the rabbit eye was clearly irritated. The phenomenon is to be investigated further.

The release of LDH is a parameter of cell membrane damage and can give additional information on the mechanism of cytotoxicity. This test showed greater intra- as well as interlaboratory variations. Differences of timing and storage seem to have an important influence on the subtle LDH release. More refined standardization procedures are being evaluated. To assess membrane leakage more closely, it would also be necessary to do kinetic analysis, whereas this study was planned as a fixed-time study.

PGE_2 detection in the medium was studied as an indicator of inflammatory mediator synthesis. Compared with the MTT_{50} quantification, PGE_2 assays showed a wider range of results within laboratories as well as between laboratories. Nevertheless, 13 out of 18 substances were identically evaluated by the four labs. For shampoos, chlorides, preservatives, and solvents, the PGE_2 synthesis correlated with irritancy, confirming this endpoint as a significant tool in the overall estimation of the potential in vivo irritancy.

18.4   Conclusions

The aim of the present study was to find a reliable and reproducible model to replace in vivo Draize ocular tests. We believe that with the Skin²™ Model ZK 1100 we have found what we have been looking for. The technical subtleties of the tissue culture assay and the quantitative determinations of MTT, LDH and PGE_2 were mastered, and the Skin²™ model proved to be stable for wide geographical distribution.

The ease and speed of handling, the multiple quantitative endpoints, and its human origin make Skin²™ an ideal model for evaluating toxicity, understanding modes of action, and assessing irritant potential in product development and safety testing.

Reference

Braa, S. S. and Triglia D. (1991) Predicting ocular irritation using 3-dimensional human fibroblast cultures. *Cosmetics and Toiletries* **106,** 5558.

19   Cellular Assays for Testing Peritoneal Dialysis Bags

Mary Dawson and Zara Jabar

Summary

The paper describes a cell culture method for testing plastic dialysis bags for toxic substances which may leak out of them into dialysis fluids. The indices of toxicity used were cellular changes as seen by microscopy, and accelerated fall in the transmonolayer resistance of cell sheets.

Abbreviations. CAPD = continuous ambulatory peritoneal dialysis; DEHP = di-2-ethylhexyl phthalate.

19.1   Introduction

Patients in terminal kidney failure are ideally treated by transplant. Unfortunately in some parts of the world this is not available, and, where it is, the number of suitable available kidneys is far short of requirements, probably mainly due to thoughtlessness on the part of the general public. The waiting time for a kidney in Britain now is about three years. Thus measures have to be instituted to keep the patient alive and as well as possible during his anxious wait.

There are two types of dialysis available for this: the type where the patient is attached for many hours to a kidney machine, and the type called continuous ambulatory peritoneal dialysis (CAPD), where he has much more freedom of movement. He is fitted with an indwelling peritoneal catheter, a short stub protruding. To this is aseptically attached by flexible tubing a bag of warmed dialysis fluid (the common inorganic ions plus glucose). This flows in by gravity. The empty bag is detached or tucked into a waistband, leaving the patient mobile for some hours, when the fluid is drained out again by gravity, and discarded, a new bag being attached. About four bags per day is usual. Bags are not re-used in Britain.

However, two serious side effects have been reported. One is the deposition of collagen and similar materials in the peritoneum (sclerosing retro-peritonitis). This may be so extensive that peristalsis is halted, with fatal outcome. The other is the failure of the peritoneal membrane to continue to act as a dialyzing membrane, which means that the treatment has to be abandoned, again with fatal outcome.

Alternatives to Animal Testing. New Ways in the Biomedical Sciences, Trends and Progress.
Reinhardt, C. A. (ed.). 1994. © VCH, Weinheim.

Naturally, various possible reasons have been adduced. These include: the nature of the disinfectant used to cleanse connectors at bag changes (dregs of it enter the peritoneum); the composition of the dialysis fluid, both in respect of original ingredients and in respect of alterations on sterilization and storage, and in respect of additives intended to prevent decomposition of the fluid; the nature of the buffer added to the solutions; infections; natural surfactant in and around the peritoneum; and substances extracted from dialysis fluid containers.

Animal experiments have in many cases been defeated both by the fact that the animals were not in terminal renal failure, and by the high mortality rates involved in trying to model CAPD in small animals.

The present work continues the authors' previous cell culture studies in this field (Jabar and Dawson, 1989a, 1989b, 1990, 1991) and specifically concerns eluate from plastic bags.

19.2   Safety of plastic bags for peritoneal dialysis fluid

Some years ago glass bottles as containers for dialysis and intravenous fluids were replaced with plastic bags. These are lighter and less fragile to transport, and do not need an air inlet to allow fluid to run out, this having always carried the risk of contamination.

However, doubts have been cast on the safety of plastics in relation to materials that might be leached out of them into their contents on storage. Problems arise for fluid manufacturers in that they buy the bags from bag manufacturers who in turn have bought them from plastic manufacturers. The bags usually consist of 55–60% polyvinyl chloride (pvc), 35–40% plasticizer (usually di-2-ethylhexyl phthalate (DEHP), together with unreacted monomer, antioxidants, lubricants (usually stearic acid and liquid paraffin), fillers to reduce costs, stabilizers (usually soaps) and pigment (usually ultramarine to mask the yellowish color). Some bags are of sophisticated construction, having an outer, more heavily plasticized layer and an inner layer less plasticized next to the fluid. However, plasticizer migration has been observed from outer to inner layers, and it appears difficult to find a suitable barrier to put between the layers. It is known that migration is greater into fatty than into aqueous contents, and increases with temperature increase above ambient. Dialysis fluids are warmed to body temperature before use. It is known also that pvc sheds particles, but that was not part of the present investigation.

Details of the composition are often not disclosed to fluid manufacturers, who therefore test each batch of bags bought to ensure that they comply with British Standards 2463 and 5736 (British Standards, 1962, 1989), or corresponding standards in other countries in which they wish to market. The standards include animal tests as follows:

– For tissue implantation tests: 3 anesthetized rabbits;
– For systemic toxicity tests: 24 mice, later killed and autopsied;
– For intracutaneous tests: 4 rabbits, using several samples per rabbit;
– For pyrogen tests: 3 rabbits, using more if results are equivocal;
– For sensitization tests: 36 guinea pigs;
– For skin irritation tests: 6 rabbits for extracts, 3 for solid devices;
– For eye tests: 3 rabbits.

To gauge how many animals altogether may be used one must know that plastics manufacturers come and go with such frequency that any one fluid manufacturer may test about 100
different plastics per year. Thus it is clearly worthwhile in terms of animal sparing to develop
a useful cell culture test.

The British Standards do in fact mention cell culture tests, but these are on only the
extracts, not on the plastics themselves, and different substances may be extracted into contents of different composition, pH value or storage temperature. Also the cell types are not
relevant to the peritoneum, and the endpoint is subjective, the cells being fixed and stained
and scored 0–4 for percentage of cell death.

Our test is based on disruption of epithelial sheets, both as seen by microscope, and as
measured by fall in transmonolayer resistance, i.e. a quantitative response, and a closer
model of the peritoneum.

19.3 Materials and methods

MDCK cells (European Collection of Animal Cell Cultures, Porton Down, England) are cultured in Ham's F12 medium (Flow Laboratories, Irvine, Scotland) with added glutamine and
containing 10 % foetal calf serum in Falcon Primaria flasks (Messrs. Beveridge, Edinburgh,
Scotland), or on Cellagen culture plate inserts, 14 mm in diameter (ICN Biomedicals, Cleve-

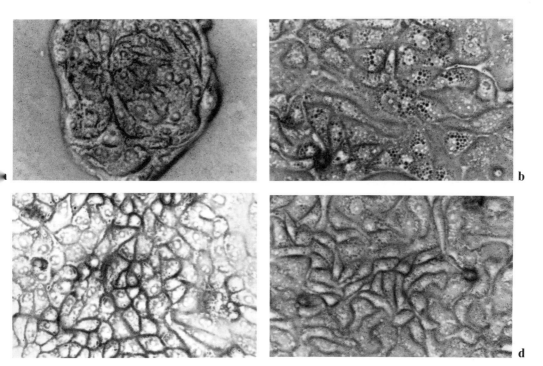

Figure 19-1. Experiments using whole plastic. Plastic added after monolayer had formed. a) Untreated cells
before monolayer had fully been formed. b) Vacuolization. c) Retraction of cells in sheet. d) Distortion of
cells in sheet.

168   M. Dawson, Z. Jabar

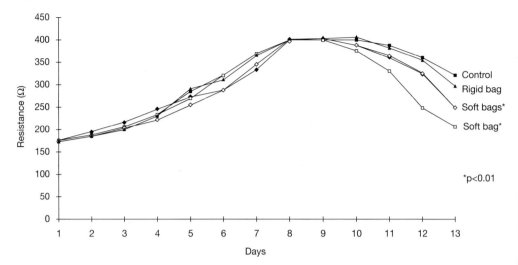

Figure 19-2. Accelerated fall in transmonolayer resistance following the addition of samples of dialysis bags to confluent MDCK cells. Resistance rises as confluency is attained. Control, without plastic, shows the natural drop as cells age. The more rigid bag showed a drop not significantly different from this by t-test. The softer bags produced results which did differ significantly from the control.

land, U.S.A.) in Cel-Cult square well culture plates (Sterilin Ltd., Feltham, England). Resistance was measured with an epithelial voltohmmeter (World Precision Instruments, New Haven, U.S.A.).

For microscopy, the cells were grown in the 25 cm² flasks, using 5 ml of medium per flask. Four pieces of bag (1 cm²) were added per flask. Before addition, they were washed several times in sterile culture medium. Because of the volume of medium, the pieces floated and did not touch the cells. Plastic was added a) with the cells to study inhibition of monolayer formation, and b) after the cell monolayer had formed, to study its disruption.

Similarly di-2-ethylhexyl phthalate (DEHP; Aldrich, Gillingham, Dorset, U.K.) was added on two analogous occasions. Each experiment consisted of 16 replicates.

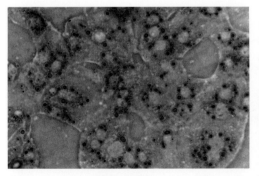
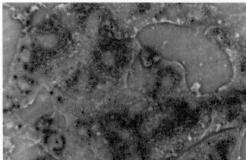

Figure 19-3. Experiments using pure plasticizer. Plasticizer added after monolayer had formed. a) Engulfed spheres of plasticizer were observed. b) Vacuolization.

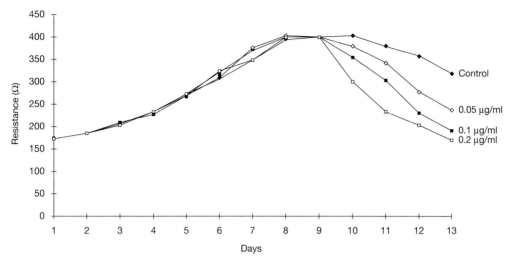

Figure 19-4. Accelerated fall in transmonolayer resistance following the addition of varying amounts of di-2-ethylhexyl phthalate to confluent MDCK cells. The fall is seen to be dose-dependent.

For the conductivity experiments, the materials were added at monolayer confluency of cells on the inserts in the wells. Each conductivity experiment consisted of 12 replicates. The use of square wells allowed the insertion of electrodes into the corners of the wells.

19.4   Results

Plastic from softer bags (presumably with more plasticizer) inhibited normal cell monolayer formation, and fibroblast-like cells were also seen among the cells. The abnormal monolayer had abnormal cell-cell adhesion. Therefore there was an absence of tight junctions, essential for normal transmonolayer transport.

When plastic was added after the monolayer had already formed, cell vacuolization, retraction and distortion took place (Figure 19-1).

Thus the material leached out from the plastic was disruptive of the cultured monolayers.

In the conductivity experiments (Figure 19-2), the plastic was added after monolayer formation. The accelerated fall in resistance caused by plastic from the three softer bags was significantly different from the controls without plastic by t-test, whereas the fall caused by plastic from the more rigid bag was not significantly different.

There are so many substances in bag plastic, as mentioned above, that it was of interest to test the plasticizer itself.

Microscopy experiments showed again inhibition of normal cell monolayer formation, and, in the case of the plasticizer added to already formed monolayers (Figure 19-3), vacuolization was again observed, and also engulfment of spheres of plasticizer.

The results of the conductivity experiments with plasticizer are shown in Figure 19-4. The plasticizer was used in doses of 0.05, 0.1, and 0.2 µg/ml, added at confluency. The loss of confluency is seen to be dose-dependent.

19.5   Discussion

There is extensive literature on the toxicity of plasticizers (Corley *et al.*, 1977; Kjellstrand and Boberg, 1991; Lee, 1987; MAFF, 1990; Petrick *et al.*, 1977; Rubin and Jaeger, 1973; Woodward, *et al.*, 1986), including comprehensive reviews.

DEHP intake has been associated with acute and long-term effects in many species including humans. Sadly, factory employees coming in contact with the materials have yielded much of the information. Some has arisen also from dialysis patients. Kidney failure patients excrete plasticizer more slowly than normal persons, and do so *via* the bile duct. However, the long-term effects of repeated doses are not yet known (Jones, 1989). Liver damage has been among the effects reported. This is important because, in addition to direct pathological changes, there could be effects also on the metabolism of most drugs.

Thus it is of the greatest importance to design a test which would enable one to find out if plasticizer is contaminating dialysis fluid. Our test is useful, not only in avoiding animal use, but also in being applicable to both whole plastic and pure plasticizer, and in being able to show a dose related response. Also, it is easily reproducible in different laboratories so that results can be validly compared.

Acknowledgements. The authors thank the Humane Research Trust for financing this work, and one of us (MD) thanks the Universities Federation for Animal Welfare for defraying the cost of presenting this paper at the SIAT Symposium.

References

British Standards (1962) British standard 2463, *BS* Part 1. (Update: British standard 1089, *BS* Part 2, 1991). Milton Keynes, U.K.

British Standards (1989) British standard 5736, *BS* Part 1. Milton Keynes, U.K.

Corley J. H., Needham T. E., Sumner E. D. and Mikeal R., (1977) Effect of various factors on the amount of plasticizer in intravenous solution packaged in flexible bags. *American Journal of Hospital Pharmacy* **34**, 259–264.

Jabar Z. and Dawson M. (1989a) The disruptive effect of reactive oxygen species (ROS) on sheets of cultured epithelia. *Journal of Pharmacy and Pharmacology* **41**, 42P.

Jabar Z. and Dawson M. (1989b) The effect of chlorhexidine on Madin Darby canine kidney cells. *Molecular Toxicology* **1**, 445–452.

Jabar Z. and Dawson M. (1990) The role of cell culture in improving continuous ambulatory peritoneal dialysis. *ATLA* **18**, 259–265.

Jabar Z. and Dawson M. (1991) The role of surfactant in continuous ambulatory peritoneal dialysis. *Toxicology in Vitro* **5**, 467–471.

Jones C. (1989) *Blood responses to plasticised poly (vinyl chloride).* Doctoral dissertation, University of Strathclyde, Glasgow.

Kjellstrand P. and Boberg U. (1991) Testing of polymer materials. What methods should be used? *ATLA* **19**, 222–225.

Lee S. M. (Editor) (1987) *Advances in Biomaterials.* Vol. 1. Technomic Publ. Co., Inc., Lancaster, PA, U.S.A.

Ministry of Agriculture, Fisheries and Food (MAFF) (1990) *Plasticisers: Continuing Surveillance. 30th Report of Steering Group on Food Surveillance* (Food Surveillance Paper No. 30). H.M.S.O., London.

Petrick R. J., Loucas S. P., Cohl J. K. and Mehl B. (1977) Review of current knowledge of plastic intravenous fluid containers. *American Journal of Hospital Pharmacy* **34**, 357–362.

Rubin R. J. and Jaeger R. J. (1973) Some pharmacologic and toxicologic effects of di-2-ethylhexyl phthalate (DEHP) and other plasticizers. *Environmental Health Perspectives* **3**, 53–59.

Woodward K. N., Smith A. M., Mariscotti S. P. and Tomlinson N. J. (1986) *Toxicity Review 14, of the Health and Safety Executive, Review of the Toxicity of the Esters and O-phthalic Acid (Phthalate Esters).* H. M. S. O., London.

20 The Position of the Authorities

Lavinia Pioda

Summary

The Swiss toxic substances legislation (1969) requires the classification of chemicals according to five categories based on their total toxicity. Whereas toxicological data are required for
the classification of basic substances, a computational method is employed for formulated
products. The provisions of the Swiss animal protection law (1981), which call for a drastic
and stepwise limitation of animal experiments, have also led to the revision of other laws.
Experience in Switzerland, with its large multinational companies, has shown that the
achievement of a genuine breakthrough for alternative methods is possible only at the international level. The introduction of alternatives also requires a rethinking of the philosophy
underlying current regulatory policy.

20.1 Introduction

When I received my doctoral degree hardly anyone had ever heard of alternative methods. It
is only recently that people have begun talking about alternatives – a fundamentally new concept, which has developed within the course of my career. At that time, enthusiasm was generated by animal testing – experimental methods which appeared to provide exact results, but
in fact did not. Quantitative data increase the feeling of security in the screening and classification of substances, because numbers are neutral and convenient for generalizing from the
results of animal experiments to the potential risk of an unknown substance for humans.

In Switzerland, there are two governmental agencies with relevance for experimental
methods using animals and alternatives: a) The Federal Veterinary Office (Bundesamt für
Veterinärwesen), which executes the animal protection law, and b) the Federal Health Office
(Bundesamt für Gesundheitswesen), which sets the standards for the evaluation and toxicity
classification of substances and is responsible for the registration of chemicals. In addition,
the Intercantonal Drug Control Bureau (IKS) is responsible for registering drugs.

The animal protection law has been in force since 1981. The following commentary on
the first decade of its implementation was made at a media conference in June 1991:

> In connection with the submission in 1986 of a popular initiative calling for the drastic
> and stepwise limitation of animal experiments as well as with numerous other occur-

Alternatives to Animal Testing. New Ways in the Biomedical Sciences, Trends and Progress.
Reinhardt, C. A. (ed.). 1994. © VCH, Weinheim.

rences, the issues surrounding animal experimentation have been subject to exhaustive public debate in the past years. Since the animal protection legislation came into effect, its impact has been increasingly felt, and it has led to better protection of animals used in experimentation without unduly limiting research. (translated from Steiger, 1992, p. 31)

It is unnecessary here to elaborate on the possibilities of conducting fewer animal experiments without limiting research in general. Briefly, effective methods include the thorough examination of proposals for animal experiments within the framework of the acceptance procedure, modifications to meet regulations on the housing and care of animals, and adherence to the concept of animal protection in connection with the Swiss registration procedure for chemicals.

20.2   The advancement of alternative methods

There has been a significant reduction in the number of animals used for experimentation in Switzerland: In 1983 two million animals were used; seven years later this number was reduced by almost 50 %. The animal protection law has also had an effect on the training of animal caretakers in facilities using laboratory animals as well as on the attitude of many researchers to animal experimentation.

The encouragement of research on alternatives to animal experiments and the establishment of a documentation service for alternatives in the Federal Veterinary Office are two additional indications of progress in this area. Between 1981 and 1991, the Swiss government spent around 2.5 million Swiss francs on alternatives (research grants, expert commissions). In this context, it has been interesting to note a change in policy over time as new developments gain acceptance.

20.3   The registration of chemicals and formulated products

The Federal Office of Health is responsible for the registration of chemicals. This involves alternatives only indirectly but not insignificantly. The toxic substances law requires that all chemical substances and products be registered before they can be placed on the market. Registration is based on the presentation of detailed documented experimental data. However, toxicological data are required only for the basic substances, i.e. the raw materials and the active ingredients, but not for the formulated products, and for this reason relatively few animal experiments are required to satisfy the toxic substances law. The situation is different for the development of pharmaceutical products, and as a result, it is in this area that most of the animal experiments in Switzerland are done.

For formulated products, the individual substances and their corresponding toxicity are calculated proportionately according to the percentage of the substance in the product. Although this procedure is strongly criticized by some toxicologists, our experience over several decades proves that this method adequately satisfies the concerns of the law.

20.4   Theoretical and experimental basis of classification

As far as the test results are concerned, it is irrelevant for those carrying out the classification whether the data were obtained through animal experiments or with alternative methods. On the basis of these (quantitative) data, the computer, with the help of classification programs, calculates the toxicity of the product to be classified. The registration is then communicated by means of a statement of permission ("Verfügung") to the applicant.

Given the 500–600 products to be classified per month, the necessity of automating this procedure is understandable. When the process was computerized 15 years ago, there was concern that those working with the system would cease thinking for themselves, and this has, in part, occurred. A computer program presents the temptation of producing a classification solely on the basis of the toxicity values of the individual components. For most products this is not a problem, but in order to avoid false classifications of complex products the program must be designed to take into account other factors than just the automated calculation. Originally, the method distinguished only between classified and unclassified substances, raw materials, and mixtures of ingredients. Later a more sophisticated procedure was created, according to which the decision was made whether or not an automatic classification could be carried out.

As already mentioned, there is no distinction made in this process between alternative methods and classical methods. However, underlying political influences do play a role, particularly those exerted by animal protection policies. The Federal Veterinary Office, for example, can exert influence through the animal protection law and other laws concerning animals, which are subordinate to it. When the toxic substances law was revised in 1983, the ominous term "LD_{50}" was deleted as a result of pressure from the Federal Veterinary Office and replaced (in Art. 4) by the phrase "a test on a few animals for the determination of the acute oral lethal dose," without any specification of test requirements or the number of animals used. This allows the Swiss authorities more freedom and the advantage of flexibility in comparison with the laws of other countries.

20.5   Classification of substances and the validation and acceptance of alternative methods

For the classification of substances according to the toxic substance class, a group of experts is provided with all available data, on the basis of which they carry out their evaluation and advise us of the result. We are free to accept all methods, as we make no specifications in this respect. We have also informed all interested groups that we accept all scientifically based methods of whatever kind, for example, structure-activity relationships, alternative methods, or purely computational methods. It must, however, lead to a result that our experts can evaluate. Despite our efforts at information, there has been no response, and the reason for this is that the chemical and pharmaceutical industry produces for other markets than just Switzerland.

The Swiss authorities would accept alternative methods, but the companies collect data by means of the specifically regulated animal experiments called for in other countries. Therefore they are not motivated to pursue an additional, alternative course just for Switzerland. This is the current state of affairs. Whatever can be done to improve the situation will have to take place at the international level. I am glad that Switzerland is a member of the OECD, which has become active in this field (see Van Looy, 1994, this volume). Recently, the problem of validation was extensively discussed in the OECD. It still takes 10 to 15 years until a method is validated, and as the methods are innumerous, the difficulties are nearly insurmountable.

Essentially, the methods would not necessarily have to be validated, but *accepted*. The LD_{50} method was never validated in the current sense, but simply accepted by most countries and incorporated without validation into their guidelines. Somewhere someone should have the courage to do the same with alternative methods. Especially now with the current network of international agreements, no producer willingly conducts two different tests when one of them is internationally accepted. Given this situation, it lies with the authorities to begin accepting, or even requiring, alternative methods as a substitute.

20.6   Outlook

In concluding, I should like to present one final thought. In comparing the present discussion on alternatives with that conducted during a workshop eight years ago (Reinhardt *et al.*, 1985) it is clear that today there are not only many more methods available, but also that the methods have become more sophisticated. It should not be forgotten that real alternatives are in essence revolutions, and revolutions cannot be incorporated into an existing structure. All our laws are based on animal experiments. Therefore it should be acknowledged that the existing structure will have to be changed before something revolutionary can be introduced. These thoughts are particularly directed at those who are involved in the preparation and revision of laws. If this revolutionary seed of new methods is so important for the classification of chemicals, then the philosophy of the law should be changed in accordance. Without this essential change, a breakthrough will never be achieved.

References

Reinhardt C. A., Bosshard E. and Schlatter C. (1985) International workshop on irritation testing of skin and mucous membranes (Kartause Ittingen). *Food and Chemical Toxicology* **23,** 135–338.
Steiger A. (1992) Auswirkungen, Probleme und künftige Entwicklungen im Tierschutz. *Swiss Vet* **2-S,** 21–24, 26–27, 29–32, 34–36.
Van Looy H. M. (1994) The OECD and international regulatory acceptance of the Three Rs. In *Alternatives to Animal Testing. New Ways in the Biomedical Sciences, Trends and Progress.* Edited by C. A. Reinhardt. pp. 13–19. VCH Verlagsgesellschaft, Weinheim.

Subject Index

Acceptance of alternative tests   18 f, 52
Akademie für Tierschutz   85
Alternatives to animal testing
  definition of   46
*Alternatives to Laboratory Animals,
  ATLA*   5 f, 23, 47 f
Animal experimentation
  approval procedure   60 f
  committees   60 f
  computerized teaching of   107 ff
  educational prerequisites   62 f
  ethical evaluation of projects   60 f
  political activism   2 ff
  regulation of   3 f
  see also Education, alternatives training
    programs
Animal suffering   57 ff
  distress rating   59, 72
Animal use   4, 8 f, 57 ff, 70 ff, 125 ff, 174
Animal welfare officer   63
Antibiotics   31, 33
Antibody production   83
  see also Monoclonal antibodies
Arthropods, blood-sucking   125 ff, 131 ff
*ATLA, see Alternatives to Laboratory
  Animals*
Audiovisual materials, *see* Computer
  programs in biomedical education
Awards
  Marchig Animal Welfare Award   46

Bacterial contamination   29 f
Benzene   147 ff
Biomedical education, computer-aided
  programs in   107 ff
Blood-brain barrier, in vitro model of   96
Blood feeding   125 ff
Bone marrow culture   147 ff, 154 f
British Standards   166 f

British Union for the Abolition of
  Vivisection   4
British Veterinary Association   47, 49 f
BUAV, *see* British Union for the
  Abolition of Vivisection
BVA, *see* British Veterinary Association

CAAT, *see* Johns Hopkins University
  Center for Alternatives to Animal
  Testing
CAD, *see* Center for Alternatives
  to Animal Testing
CADD, *see* Computer-aided drug design
Carbonic anhydrase, model for   101 ff
Carnation test   28 f, 35 f
Cell culture
  bone marrow   147 ff
  genetically engineered cells   81
  hepatocytes, and co-cultures   141 ff,
    147 ff
  MDCK cells, monolayer   167 ff
  perifusion system   141 ff
  reaggregate cultures   93 ff
  see also In vitro test
Cellular functions
  albumin assay   150
  ATP depletion   36
  basal   36
  cell growth   151 f
  cell stress   81, 96
  cell viability   36, 150 f, 155
  hypoxia   36
  transepithelial resistance   168 f
Center for Alternatives to Animal Testing
  (Netherlands)   67 ff
Center for Documentation and Evaluation
  of Alternative Methods to Animal
  Experiments (Germany), *see* ZEBET
Charles University, Hradec Krßlov   120 ff

CHEN assay, *see* Chick embryo neural
   cell assay
Chick embryo neural cell assay   93 ff
Classification of substances   175 f
Coagulation process   30 ff
COLIPA   23, 53, 82
Committee for the Reform of Animal
   Experimentation (U.K.)   47, 49 f
Computer-aided drug design   99 ff
   Computer-aided teaching and animal
   experimentation   107 ff
   interactivity   111
   pedagogical value of   108 f
Computer programs
   in biomedical education
      computer controlled mannequins
         114 f
      courseware   111 ff
      interactive video   113 ff
      pharmacology   109 ff
      physiology   109 ff
      software   109 ff
      virtual reality   115 f
   for molecular interaction   101 ff
Conductivity of epithelial monolayers
   167 ff
Cosmetic, Toiletry & Fragrance
   Association   7, 52
Cosmetic, Toiletry & Perfumery
   Association   53
Cosmetics, cruelty free   53
Cosmetics testing   159 ff
CRAE, *see* Committee for the Reform of
   Animal Experimentation
Cryopreservation   132, 134 ff
CTFA, *see* Cosmetic, Toiletry &
   Fragrance Association
CTPA, *see* Cosmetic, Toiletry &
   Perfumery Association
Cyclophosphamide   147 ff
Cytochrome P450   142 f, 150 f, 154
   assay   150
Cytokines   29 f
Cytotoxicity   36, 51, 147 f, 151 f, 155,
   160 ff
   see also Toxicity testing
Czech Republic   119 ff

Databank   79, 85 ff
   description of   85 ff

Galileo Data Bank   23, 79
Gelbe Liste   79, 85 ff
in vitro toxicology databanks   79
INVITTOX   23, 52, 79
PREX   63 f
users of   88
ZEBET databank   77 ff
see also Information services for alter-
   natives
DG XI of the EC   80, 82
DG XII of the EC   80
Disseminated intravascular coagulation
   30, 32, 36
Documentation on alternatives,
   see Databank
Draize eye irritation test   161, 163
   alternatives validation study   52, 81 f,
      159 ff
   Draize test campaign   7 f
Drug metabolism   141 ff, 147 ff
Drug screening   99 ff

Eastern Europe, alternatives in
   German Democratic Republic   82 f
   Czech Republic   120 ff
ECETOC   17, 23
ECITTS   24, 52, 92
ECVAM, *see* European Center for the
   Validation of Alternative Methods
Education
   alternatives training programs   24,
      61 ff, 120 ff
      EC TEMPUS JEP   49, 119 ff
      lack of   91
      see also Animal experimentation
   computer-aided programs in   107 ff
   FRAME   49
EFPIA   23
Emulation software   111
   PharmaTutor program   111, 113
Endothelial cells   30
Endotoxic shock   27 ff
Endotoxin   29 ff
   disseminated intravascular coagulation
      30
   endothelial cells   30
   standard   32, 37
Endpoints   36 f
   LAL test   34, 37
   Skin^2 model   160

ERGATT, *see* European Research Group
  for Alternatives in Toxicity Testing
Ethical principles   2
Ethics committee   60 f
Ethoxycoumarin O-deethylase (ECOD)
  activity   142 ff
EUROGROUP for Animal Welfare   23
European Centre for the Validation of
  Alternative Methods   21 ff, 52
  activities   23 f
  development of alternatives   22 ff
  information services   23
European Community
  Commission of the   21 ff
  Council of the   21 f
European Parliament   21 f
European Research Group for Alternatives
  in Toxicity Testing   7, 23, 51 f, 92

FDA guideline   31 ff
Feeding, artificial membrane technique
  126 ff
Filarial parasite research
  artificial feeding in   125 ff, 132 ff
  cryopreservation in   132, 134 ff
  in vitro cultivation of parasite stages
    134, 136 f
  maintenance of filarial cycles   125 ff,
    131 ff
  reduction of laboratory animals in
    125 ff, 131 ff
Fixed dose procedure   17 f
FRAME   4 ff, 23, 36, 45 ff, 120 ff
  education   49
  publications   47 f, 51
  Research Programme   51
  Toxicity Committee   49
The Free University of Berlin   120 ff
Fund for the Replacement of Animals in
  Medical Experiments, *see* FRAME
Funding of alternatives   6 ff, 51, 60, 71,
  80 f, 174
    criteria for   80

Galileo Data Bank   23, 79
Gelbe Liste   79, 85 ff
GLP (Good Laboratory Practice)   16
German Animal Welfare Association
  databank   85 ff
Governmental authorities, and acceptance
  of alternatives   175 f

Hematopoiesis   147 f, 151 f, 154 ff
Hepatocytes, *see* Cell culture
HET-CAM test   82
Horseshoe crab   32
Humane Society of the United States   5

IACUCs (U.S.A.)   9 f
Information services for alternatives
  ECVAM   23
  Swiss Federal Veterinary Office   91,
    174
  ZEBET   75 ff
  see also Databank
Institute linked center for alternatives
  69 ff
Insulin batch testing   9
In vitro maintenance of parasite stages
  132 ff
In vitro test   27 ff
  acceptance   29, 36 f
  albumin assay   150
  calcitonin   81
  CHEN test   93 ff
  conductivity   167 ffj
  cytochrome P450   150
  development of   27 ff, 92 ff
    strategies for   27 ff
  in insulin testing   9
  LAL test
    evolution of   34 f
    limitations of   33, 35
    validation of   33, 36 f
  LDH assay   160 f
  MTT assay   160 f
  NTE assay   96
  porphyrins   87
  in vaccine testing   72 ff, 81
  viability assay   150 f
  see also Cell culture
In vitro vs. in vivo comparison   31 f, 81 f,
  96, 143 ff, 159 ff
INVITTOX databank   23, 52, 79
In vivo tests, *see* OECD guidelines,
  Draize eye irritation test
Irritancy testing, *see* Draize test, Skin²
  model

Johns Hopkins University Center for
  Alternatives to Animal Testing   7
Joint European Project   120 ff
Joint Research Centre, Environment
  Institute, Ispra   22

Laboratory animals
  animal husbandry   62 ff
  for blood feeding   125 ff
  computer programs as alternative to
    107 ff
LAL *see* Limulus amebocyte lysate test
LD$_{50}$ 18, 76, 175 f
  see also OECD guidelines 401–404
LDH release assay   160 f, 164
Legislation
  Council of Europe
    Resolution 621   5 f
  Denmark   6
  EC   21, 68
    6th Amendment   14
    EEC Cosmetics Directive (76/768),
      53
    EEC Directive (86/609)   6, 50, 75,
      119
  Germany   6, 75
  Japan
    Japanese Chemical Substances
      Control Law   14
  Netherlands
    Animal Protection Law   5 f
    Experiments on Animals Act   58 f,
      61
    Experiments on Animals Decree
      62 ff
  Sweden   6
  Switzerland   6, 91
    Animal Protection Law   91, 173 f
    Toxic Substances Law   14, 173 ff
  U.K.   49 f
    Animal Procedures Committee   50 f
    Animals (Scientific Procedures) Act
      6, 50 f
    Cruelty to Animals Act   3 f, 47, 49 f
  U.S.A.
    Animal Welfare Act Amendments   7
    Health Research Extension Act   7
    Research Modernization Act   6
    Toxic Substances Control Act   14
Lethality, animal   36
Limitations
  of animal tests   31
    pyrogenicity   31
  of LAL test   33, 35
Limulus amebocyte lysate test (LAL)
  27 ff
    applications of   33
    evolution   34 f
    FDA guideline   33, 35
    mechanisms   33
    validation of   33, 36
Littlewood Committee   4, 9
Liver cell culture   149 ff
Lonazolac   143 ff
Lord Dowding Fund   4

Mechanisms
  of LAL test   34 f
  defined endpoints   37
Medical education, alternatives in   120 ff
MEIC, *see* Multicenter Evaluation of In
  Vitro Cytotoxicity
Molecular modeling   100 f
Monoclonal antibodies   71
  see also Antibody production
MTT assay   155, 160 f
Multicenter Evaluation of In Vitro
  Cytotoxicity   36
National AntiVivisection Society (U.K.)
  4
National Institute of Public Health and
  Environmental Protection (Netherlands)
  67 f, 70 ff
NAVS, *see* National AntiVivisection
  Society (U.K.)
NCA, *see* Netherlands Centre for Alter-
  natives to Animal Experiments
Netherlands Centre for Alternatives to
  Animal Experiments   60
Neuroteratology, in vitro   92 ff
Neurotoxicity, in vitro monitoring of   95

OECD   7, 13 ff
  national coordinators   14 f
OECD guidelines
  development of   14 ff
  Guideline 401 (acute oral)   17 f
    see also LD$_{50}$
  Guideline 402 (acute dermal)   17
    see also LD$_{50}$
  Guideline 404 (acute dermal irritation/
    corrosion)   17 f
    see also LD$_{50}$
  Guideline 405 (acute eye irritation/
    corrosion)   17, 82, 160
  Guideline 406 (skin sensitization)   18

Guidelines 418, 419 (delayed neuro-
    toxicity testing) 96
Guideline 420 (fixed dose procedure)
    17 f

Parasitology, *see* Filarial parasite research
Perifusion system for cell cultures 141 ff
Pharmacopoeia, European 72 f
Photoirritancy 82
Plasticizer (DEHP) 166 f
Plastics, toxicity testing of 165 ff
Platform for Alternatives to Animal
    Experiments (Netherlands) 59 f
Potency test, *see* Vaccine testing, quality
    control of
Primates, nonhuman 50 f
Prostaglandin E2 (PGE2) assay 160 f,
    164
Pyrogenicity 29 ff
    rabbit test 27 ff

Rabbit
    Draize test 7, 161 ff
    pyrogenicity test 31 ff
Radiopharmaceuticals 31, 33
Receptor binding 99 ff
Receptor modeling 100 ff
Reduction 9, 18, 53, 71 ff, 107, 125 ff,
    131 ff
    see also Three Rs
Refinement 9 f, 18, 53, 61 ff, 71 ff
    see also Three Rs
Registration of chemicals 174
Regulatory authorities
    flexibility of 175 f
    harmonization of tests 16
    mutual acceptance of data 17, 175 f
    test acceptance requirements 13 ff,
        175 f
        for in vitro tests 37
Replacement 18, 54, 71 ff, 100, 105, 107,
    125 ff, 131 ff
    see also Three Rs
Research projects 51, 71, 81, 83
    see also Filarial parasite research
Risk assessment 29, 35 f
    see also Safety testing, Toxicity testing
RIVM, *see* National Institute of Public
    health and Environmental Protection
Rockefeller University 7

Rodent models of filariasis 131 ff
Royal Society for the Prevention of
    Cruelty to Animals 50
RSPCA, *see* Royal Society for the Preven-
    tion of Cruelty to Animals
Russell and Burch 1 ff, 10, 46, 83

Safety testing 14
    of dialysis bags 165 ff
    see also Risk assessment, Toxicity
        testing
Scottish Society for the Prevention of
    Vivisection 4
Screening 19, 92, 99 ff
Sensitivity
    of animal tests 31
    of LAL test 32
Serology 73
SIAT 89 ff
    Computer-Aided Drug Design Group
        90, 99 ff
    education 91
    In Vitro Toxicology Group 90, 92 ff
    research program 92 ff
Simulation software 109 f
    cardiac physiology model 112
    PharMACokinetix model 110
    Stella Diabetes Dynamics simulation
        109
Singer, Peter 7
Skin² model ZK1100 160 ff
    comparison with Draize test 163 f
    interlaboratory evaluation of 159 f,
        162 ff
Societies for in vitro toxicology 48
Spira, Henry 7 f
SSPV, *see* Scottish Society for the
    Prevention of Vivisection
Standardization of tests 37
Sulfonamide inhibitors 104
Swiss Institute for Alternatives to Animal
    Testing, *see* SIAT

TEMPUS program 119 ff
Three Rs
    acceptance of 13 ff, 78
        role of regulatory authorities in
            175 f
    campaigning for 45 ff
    concept of 2, 53 f, 69 f

development of, conditions for   68 ff
history of   1 ff
introduction in Czech Republic   120 ff
resistance to   8, 46, 68 ff, 175 f
revolutionary character of   176
see also Replacement, Reduction,
    Refinement
Toxicity classification of substances
    174 f
and acceptance of alternative methods
    175 f
Toxicity testing   16 ff
cosmetics   53, 81 f, 159 ff
endotoxin   29 ff
in vitro   23 f, 31 ff, 51, 81, 89 ff
neuroteratology   92 ff
organophosphates   96
plasticizers   166 ff
see also Cellular functions, cell stress,
    Cytotoxicity, Risk assessment, Safety
    testing, Validation
Toxin binding inhibition test (ToBI)   73 f

U.K. Home Office   49 f
Universities Federation for Animal
    Welfare   2 f
University of Nottingham   120 ff
U.S. Congress Office of Technology
    Assessment Report   48
U.S. Soap & Detergent Association   52

Vaccine testing   9
alternatives in   72 ff
quality control of   67 ff, 72 ff
Validation   18 f, 28 f, 101 f
Amden workshop   52, 82, 92
Draize test   81 f, 159 ff
LAL test   32 ff
photoirritancy   82
projects
    documentation of   78
    ECITTS   24, 52, 93
    ECVAM   24
    FRAME   52
    RIVM CAD   71 f
    SIAT   92
    ZEBET   81 f
strategies   52
    confidence building   18
    empirical approach   28
    heuristic/mechanistic approach   28
    pragmatic approach   18
    scientific approach   18
see also Toxicity testing
Variability, of animal tests   31

WHO guidelines   72 f

Yak computer program   101 ff

Zbinden and Flury-Roversi   7
ZEBET   75 ff, 120 ff